AIDS:
Rights, Risk and Reason

Social Aspects of AIDS

Series Editor: Peter Aggleton
Goldsmiths' College, University of London

AIDS is not simply a concern for scientists, doctors and medical researchers, it has important social dimensions too. These include cultural, individual and media responses to HIV/AIDS, stigmatization and discrimination, perceptions of risk, and issues to do with counselling, care and health promotion.

This new series of books brings together work from many disciplines including psychology, sociology, cultural and media studies, anthropology, education and history. Many of the titles offer insight into contemporary research priorities and identify some of the opportunities open to those involved in care and health promotion. The series will be of interest to the general reader, those involved in education and social research, as well as scientific and medical researchers who want to examine the social aspects of AIDS.

AIDS:
Rights, Risk and Reason

Edited by

Peter Aggleton, Peter Davies and Graham Hart

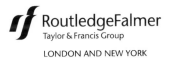

RoutledgeFalmer
Taylor & Francis Group

LONDON AND NEW YORK

First published in 1992
By Falmer Press
Reprinted 2003
By RoutledgeFalmer
11 New Fetter Lane, London EC4P 4EE

Transferred to Digital Printing 2003

A catalogue record for this book is available from the British Library

ISBN 0 75070 039 4
ISBN 0 75070 040 8 pbk

Jacket design by Caroline Archer
Typeset in 9.5/11pt Bembo by
Graphicraft Typesetters Ltd., Hong Kong
Printed and Bound by Antony Rowe Ltd

Contents

Contents

Preface

In March 1991 the Fifth Conference on Social Aspects of AIDS took place at South Bank Polytechnic in London. As in previous years, the conference attracted social researchers working in the field of health, as well as health providers in statutory and non-governmental organizations. Themes examined included perceptions of risk and risk-taking behaviour, rights and responsibilities, and the 'rationality' that underpins individual and collective responses to HIV/AIDS.

This book, like its predecessors (*Social Aspects of AIDS*, Falmer Press, 1988; *AIDS: Social Representations and Social Practices*, Falmer Press, 1989; *AIDS: Individual, Cultural and Policy Dimensions*, Falmer Press, 1990; and *AIDS: Responses, Interventions and Care*, Falmer Press, 1991), contains many of the papers given at the conference. Collectively, they demonstrate the important work that is currently underway as well as the scope of contemporary enquiry.

As editors, it has been again our privilege to work with contributors both before and after the conference. Our thanks go to Paul Broderick, Theo Blackmore, Phillip Gatter, Andrew Hunt, Ford Hickson, Heather Jones, Vijay Kumari, Michael Stephens and Peter Weatherburn for pre-conference publicity and conference administration. The Economic and Social Research Council (ESRC) provided financial support for the meeting. Finally, we must thank Sue Graham and Helen Thomas who prepared the manuscript for publication.

Peter Aggleton
Peter Davies
Graham Hart

1   Gay Men, HIV/AIDS and Social Research: An Antipodean Perspective

Gary Dowsett, Mark Davis and Bob Connell

Australia has experienced 2381 cases of AIDS as at 31 December 1990, 60 per cent of whom have died (National Centre in HIV Epidemiology and Clinical Research, 1991). Males account for 97 per cent of cases. The incidence of AIDS is still increasing in Australia, but at a slower rate than in earlier years of the epidemic. Along with New Zealand, the pattern of the Australian epidemic is different from the rest of the Western Pacific, in that the proportion of AIDS cases related to sexual transmission of the virus between men is high, 87 per cent, and has remained so since 1986.

The extent of HIV infection is far harder to gauge. Our best estimate of the number of infected Australians (December 1990) is 13,569, although the real figure could be as high as 15,000 (Solomon and Wilson, 1990; National Centre in HIV Epidemiology and Clinical Research, 1991). Figures for 1990 for New South Wales (NSW), the largest state, are not yet available, but in the other states there were 583 newly diagnosed cases of HIV infection in 1990, 66 per cent of which were related to sex between men. In these states, heterosexual transmission accounted for 2.5 per cent of overall infections, and non-homosexual drug injection for 2.9 per cent. However, one should note the high figure of 11.7 per cent for the 'Other' or undetermined category.

NSW is disproportionately affected by the epidemic and accounts for 63 per cent of national AIDS cases and 66 per cent of national HIV infections, a rate roughly three times higher than the rest of the country. Yet even these figures mask the fact that the Australian epidemic is city-based: Sydney, with a population of 3.5 million, has well over 50 per cent of the national AIDS case load. Two inner-Sydney health areas in themselves, Eastern Suburbs and Central Sydney, account for 68 per cent of New South Wales AIDS cases.

Sydney is also the site of Australia's largest gay community, and it has been very heavily hit by the epidemic. The oldest prospective study of inner-Sydney gay men found that 39 per cent of men were HIV seropositive in 1985. This figure grew to 49 per cent by 1989, although the seroconversion rate had dropped from 8 per cent per annum to less than half a per cent per annum (Burcham *et al.*, 1989). It is unlikely, however, that this is an accurate reflection of the extent of infection among Sydney's gay community.

In its first study of gay and bisexual men in New South Wales, the Social Aspects of the Prevention of AIDS (SAPA) project, based at Macquarie University in Sydney, found that 68 per cent of respondents had been tested and 25 per cent of those tested were positive. This was in 1987 (Rodden, 1990). Rates were much lower in other Australian cities such as Melbourne 16.4 per cent; Brisbane 7.2 per cent and Canberra 4.8 per cent (Campbell *et al.*, 1988; Frazer *et al.*, 1988; Kippax *et al.*, 1989). Earlier this year a small subsample of men from the original study was resurveyed; 88 per cent have now been tested and 19 per cent of those tested were positive.[1] Of those who were seropositive, three-quarters lived in the inner-Sydney area. These results are only a rough guide; but they do indicate the scale of the impact of the epidemic on the inner-Sydney gay community.

The Macquarie AIDS Research Unit: Research Programme

The original SAPA project was developed in 1986, in conjunction with the Sydney gay community, to investigate the effects of the epidemic on gay and bisexual men. Subsequent projects have developed from the original survey, known as SAPA Study A (see Dowsett, 1991, for a full discussion). These have now become part of the research programme of the recently formed Macquarie University AIDS Research Unit which is funded by the Australian Government as part of a new National Centre for HIV Social Research. This is the third such centre — the others are in Virology, and in Epidemiology and Clinical Research, both established in 1986 — and represents a belated recognition that social research has lacked much-needed coordination and infrastructure. The units of the social research centre operate individual programmes under three headings: Basic Research Studies, Baseline Studies, and Policy and Evaluation Studies. This framework was devised to capture the different contributions offered by social science and the humanities, and to address government needs for social research advice on national AIDS strategy.

The Australian National AIDS Strategy institutionalizes a cooperative approach at all levels to fight the epidemic (Commonwealth of Australia, 1989). This cooperation extends to the national policy advisory body, the Australian National Council on AIDS, which contains members drawn from gay community organizations, injecting drug-user groups, medical and non-medical academics and researchers, public health officials and, after some pressure, a person living with HIV/AIDS. The politics of HIV/AIDS are complex in a federal system like Australia, and the strategy is the product of significant struggle and negotiation, but it is within this cooperative environment that we undertake our research programme.

Basic Research Studies

Basic Research Studies are theoretically informed investigations of the psychological and social processes underlying the responses of Australians to the epidemic, both as individuals and as members of collectivities. Basic Research Studies also investigate issues where baseline methodologies are inappropriate or unsuccessful. They look at emerging issues which require 'cutting edge' approaches, and offer a critical gaze on the national response, ensuring that both immediate and longer-term issues are analyzed.

At Macquarie five basic research projects are in progress: (1) a second stage of the original study called SAPA Study B; (2) the Class, Homosexuality and AIDS Prevention (CHAP) project; (3) the Bisexual Outreach Project; (4) the Heterosexual Men and Women and Safe Sex Negotiation Study and (5) a new media project.

Baseline Studies

Baseline Studies are those which regularly describe the national situation in terms of protective and risk behaviours, behaviour change, the effectiveness of prevention, and the non-medical impact of HIV infection — a much neglected issue. These studies mostly use standard survey methods.

We currently have two baseline studies: (1) the 1991 Triple S (Sustaining Safe Sex) survey of gay and bisexual men and (2) an annual survey of over 3000 first-year university students on a number of campuses, called Behavioural Research on AIDS and Tertiary Students (BRATS). There are plans to extend these two projects nationally over the next two years. Future plans include a new Sydney gay and bisexual men's cohort and a feasibility study for a national benchmark survey of high-risk behaviours, to be undertaken with colleagues in the other units and another national centre.

Policy and Evaluation Studies

In Policy and Evaluation Studies at Macquarie we have just completed a critical review of Australia's national media education campaigns for the Commonwealth Government. We are just about to start a new study on discrimination, leading to the development of a national benchmark survey. Other such work includes providing research advice on the latest national education campaign, designing the evaluation process for the NSW Government's Non-English-Speaking Communities AIDS Education Project, and a close-focus study of functional injecting drug users in connection with the NSW AIDS Bureau.

It is envisaged that the new centre will provide policy and evaluation advice to the government and non-government sectors by a process of consultancy work and commissioned research.

Collaborative Research

It is a key element of our approach to work collaboratively with HIV/AIDS educators, policy-makers and other researchers. This is one way to ensure that our research is useful, on target and responsive to real needs. Sometimes we succeed in this and sometimes we do not. Sometimes we are too slow and events pass us by, while at other times we find it difficult to convince our collaborators of our findings. We have also had to devise better ways to inform our audience of our findings.

One important collaborative relationship is that with the AIDS Council of NSW (ACON), the largest gay community HIV/AIDS service organization in Australia with over seventy staff and a budget of A.$4.4 million, most of which comes from the NSW and Commonwealth governments. We also provide research and policy advice to other community organizations around Australia. This collaborative principle has been incorporated into the programme of the new national centre.

The Sydney gay community has responded remarkably to this epidemic through ACON and its other organizations (Dowsett, 1990). Its efforts at prevention have been successful in achieving significant sexual behaviour change.

Gay Community Responses: The SAPA Project

The original research project, SAPA Study A, was a survey of men in NSW who have sex with men, undertaken during the southern hemisphere summer of 1986–87.[2] Five hundred and thirty five men were interviewed by twenty-five field workers, with a questionnaire which covered knowledge of HIV transmission, sexual relations and practices, social aspects of gay community life, exposure to education programmes and materials, and other health related issues (Connell *et al.*, 1988).

The survey confirmed the success of the gay communities' education strategies: gay men report these as their major sources of information and clearly use that information in changing their sexual behaviour (Kippax *et al.*, 1990). Considerable sexual behaviour change has occurred, and successful change is significantly related to attachment to organized gay communities (see Chapter 8, this volume). It is important to note, however, that less economically and sexually secure men, whose circumstances make male-to-male sex difficult to explore, have achieved less effective behaviour change (Connell *et al.*, 1989).

Overall, our findings point to *informed social support* as a vital ingredient in a *collective* response to the epidemic. This response works on two levels: the gay community organizations have worked hard to create a *safe-sex culture*, utilizing the idea of a community acting to protect itself; there is also an interpersonal dimension whereby gay men are providing information, support and encouragement to each other.

Gay community educators and researchers were encouraged by these findings, but beyond them other questions emerged. What was the sexual context in which these changes were made? The impact of social class was revealed in subtle ways in the data. What did that mean? Can such behaviour change be sustained? Who was still practising unsafe sex, and why? It was clear that achieving safe sex was more than just an individual decision; it was a collective or social process. How were we to investigate these more complex issues once the counting had been done?

We had designed the survey to answer some of these questions. We found that in NSW, as elsewhere, unprotected anal sex was more common within regular relationships than in casual encounters (Connell *et al.*, 1990). It is clear that anal intercourse, though highly physically and emotionally satisfying, was practised by only about half the men in the sample. Oral sex, a touch less physically and somewhat less emotionally satisfactory, was practised almost universally among gay men, along with mutual masturbation, kissing and massage.

Further analysis pointed to a patterning of the homosexual repertoire (Connell and Kippax, 1990). Gay sex is capable of being grouped into three repertoires differentially practised by men; a group of *oral/tactile*, 'safe' practices including oral sex, engaged in by almost all gay men; a second group, focused on *anal* sex in various forms, excluding fisting, practised with varying frequency by about 50 per cent of gay men; and the third group we called *esoteric* practices, which includes fisting, SM and watersports, and practised by less than 10 per cent of men.

These findings offer a complex picture of homosexual desire. The range of sexual practices is diverse, and sodomy is less obvious in gay sexual practice than in the public mind. Penetrative sex is nonetheless important and some men *state* a preference for the insertive or receptive mode; but in practice gay sex is commonly reciprocal. There was a strong sense that gay men consciously choose to forego pleasurable activity in order to pleasure others and also remain safe from HIV infection.

This survey is one of the major studies of gay and bisexual men in Australia. It is widely cited and has been influential in helping shape education programmes for gay and bisexual men. The project received a 1990 AIDS Trust of Australia award for its contribution to HIV/AIDS research. We are justly proud of that award, because it marks one of only two occasions in Australia when a non-medical contribution to research on HIV/AIDS has been recognized.

New Research on Gay and Bisexual Men

SAPA Study B grew out of the findings of the survey, Study A, and investigates in depth the sexual and social responses of gay-identified men to the epidemic, through case studies developed from lengthy, semi-structured, audio-recorded interviews.

It addresses the following issues: sustaining safe sex; gay community; class.

Sustaining Safe Sex

Peter is a professional man, gay-identified and living in the heart of the inner-Sydney gay quarter, known as 'Oxford Street'; it was he who first alerted us in 1987 to the difficulties some gay men were having with safe sex. In the survey Peter was what we called a 'safe sex exemplar': he achieved a score well above average on his knowledge of what was 'unsafe' with reference to HIV transmission, although he scored lower than average on his knowledge of what was 'safe'. He had engaged in only a limited range of safe sexual practices within the previous six months and had close personal experience of the epidemic. Furthermore, as an untested person, he appeared to be a success story for HIV/AIDS education.

When he was interviewed a year later, Peter was in difficulty. His low scores on what was 'safe' in gay sex actually translated into such a restricted sexual repertoire that he was fast becoming sexually and emotionally dysfunctional. He had been unable to pursue any new relationships, and sex was confined to a small number of casual encounters in sex-on-premises venues. In these, only mutual masturbation occurred; no kissing, no oral sex, and no anal sex with or without condoms. But on one or two occasions he had allowed casual sexual partners to fellate him and he ejaculated into their mouths — a practice Peter rates as unsafe.

Some of the tension of living with the epidemic is revealed by this example. If an educated, sexually sophisticated man was having difficulty in sustaining safe sex, what was happening for others, particularly those less well-educated, who lived further away from Oxford Street, and who scored less well on our knowledge and practice survey items?

Our research in Canberra, the national capital, found highly educated men's responses to safe sex to be far more complex than the basic educational messages given out by gay community prevention campaigns (Kippax *et al.*, 1989). More recent work in Australia has also confirmed that gay men are adopting many different strategies to deal with sex within relationships (Vadasz and Lipp, 1990). These findings point to new dilemmas for preventive education. Other men revealed different facets of the problem. James, in his mid-50s, nursed his infected lover for a number of years until the latter's death last year, without once breaking safe sex rules — a none too easy task. Cecil, having left a wife and family at age 53 to 'come out', was only practising safe sex. But he corrected us firmly for talking about young gay men's problems with safe sex, and indicated that being newly sexual is not just a problem for the young, and learning safe sex is just as difficult for older men too.

There has been little work done on the adoption of safe sex which goes beyond the correlates of behaviour change. In our concern to quantify the epidemic, we often overlook the deep emotional and sexual dilemmas of gay men as they struggle with avoiding or giving up sexual practices which are deeply cathected. Few heterosexual men could easily give up vaginal intercourse and, although some women may be less troubled at the prospect, neither will be asked to do so in the name of prevention.

These gay men indicate that understanding safe sex, incorporating it into a sexual repertoire and sustaining that change is a difficult process. Safe sex is something which has to be worked at continually; decisions are undermined by circumstances and by the not always obvious operation of desire. Difficulty in sustaining safe sex is not adequately described by simplistic ideas like 'addiction', or in terms like 'relapse'. Relapse is often defined as a return to or a falling back into an illness or wrongdoing. For homosexual men, anal sex is neither illness nor wrongdoing. It just assists in transmitting a virus at this moment in history. No one would ever use the term 'relapse' for heterosexuals who engage in vaginal intercourse without condoms (either in the face of HIV/AIDS or as an issue of contraception) or describe them as ill or wrongdoers. A barely disguised homophobia underlies the use of these terms for gay men struggling with this epidemic for the past seven to ten years.

Difficulties in sustaining safe sex have certainly led to new HIV infections. Barney, also in his mid-50s and a self-employed electrician, found out he was seropositive between the survey and the interview. He talked inaccurately of the 'window period', but later suggested that the insertive partner was unlikely to become infected. Barry, a seropositive teacher, said he believed that casual partners who suggested an unsafe practice were probably positive. In the absence of a strategy to verify this, Barry knows he has infected at least one man. Martin, a heterosexually-identified, bisexual man in his late 40s, still believed in early 1989 that women could not get HIV. While he had stopped unprotected anal sex with men, he was not using condoms with women.

It is clear that education about HIV transmission is an ongoing task. We need continuous information programmes for those ignorant of the issues, for those who are yet to be reached, and for those who only partially understand. In addition, sustaining safe sex also requires substantial ongoing support and education based on a more complex conceptualization of sexual desire. Research needs to pursue more sophisticated analyses of the problem of sustaining safe sex than quantifying and correlating it. Sex is not a simple act of cognition, open to scrutiny by checklist; it is a deeply complex experience, historically structured and culturally specific, often approached with incomprehension and even ambivalence. Sexual behaviour change is a *social* dilemma, the solution to which will not be found by research which seeks merely to construct those in difficulty as problem individuals.

Gay Community

Successful HIV prevention measures call for strategies of gay community development. Indeed, some of the argument for homosexual law reform in Australia has been couched in terms of facilitating gay community contributions to prevention. The fact that three states have decriminalized male homosexuality during the epidemic is a public recognition of the success of gay communities in their HIV/AIDS work. This recognition contrasts sharply with the cruel attempt in Britain to recriminalize consensual homosexual sex in recent proposed legislation.

Yet we see little research on the gay community as a community. Where are the studies of the impact of HIV infection on gay communities, on the relationships, rituals and institutions which give meaning to gay community life, on the cumulative effects of loss on a generation of men? Only one small study has ever touched on this issue in Australia.[3] Why are community health experts, community education academics and community studies researchers uninterested in this issue?

Class

SAPA Study A also revealed that men with fewer years of education, in lower-status occupations and with lower incomes were not faring so well. These data led to a second study, the CHAP project, in which we work closely with ACON in particular with its outreach and youth projects and a branch in a nearby provincial city.[4]

Huey, aged 39, has been making sandwiches on shift work for nine years. He is no fool, but an intelligent and amusing commentator on gay life. Huey, as Harriet, is also a well-known drag artiste. Huey gets plenty of sex, most of it in public toilets, and as a reporter on the sexual rituals of 'beats', as we call them in Australia, he is an ethnographer's delight. As Harriet, he used to get lots of sex — mainly with heterosexual men who liked 'dragons' (drag queens) while working as a transsexual prostitute. He is HIV seronegative and started using condoms for all anal and oral sex in the early 1980s when he first heard of AIDS. Like most sex workers in Australia, his reaction to the epidemic has been very responsible. Huey started sex with other boys at a very young age, like many other working-class men we spoke with.

Another man, Richard, had his first affair at 12 and it lasted three years. By his late teens he was working in the hospitality industry — an employment haven for working-class gays — and exploring fully gay life in Sydney, and eventually London, New York and Amsterdam. Yet he developed few longstanding friendships and now, with AIDS, is being nursed by his parents back home, angry and embittered, a reluctant participant in a provincial scene.

Chris, once top man in the leather/SM set, is now so overwhelmed by the deaths of friends that he has withdrawn to his two-room flat surrounded by fading memorabilia and framed postcards of gorgeous younger men. Chris' social life now consists of occasional dinners with a clutch of fading 'queens', a far cry from the heavy 'macho' scene of a few years ago. He was a country lad who came to the city for a career and to be gay. He has worked since in a lowly paid clerical position, only marginally more secure than Huey and Richard's jobs. His failure to succeed has a lot to do with class and sexuality issues, issues we are still exploring.

Paul has engaged in some part-time prostitution, a little heroin, a few confused relationships, and now, after a serious physical assault on account of his being gay, is awaiting compensation from a lengthy court case. Unable to work and frustrated, he fears the increasing allure of drug use. At 24, after ten years of homosexual sex, Paul has still not found a gay 'place'.

These men tell of another gayness, one informed by their experience of social inequality, low incomes and sometimes poverty, and labour market instability. These men are very different from each other but they are all gay community-identified men. Huey is a tireless fundraiser for HIV/AIDS, particularly as the more glamorous Harriet. Richard, getting thinner by the day, faithfully wears his 501s, a beard and check shirts, every inch a clone from the 70s. Chris — imposing in leather, meek out of it — built up the Sydney SM scene in the 1970s.

They are also linked by their attachment to gay life. There is an almost brittle determination in Richard to be at the heart of modern gay life. Yet he certainly hates his provincial gay scene, distinctly lacking in glamour, full as it is of drag queens, of sweet youths in love with each other, and a history of closetry. Neither Huey, unsuccessful in sex outside beats, nor Harriet, never short of an offer, has a place in the gay venues of Sydney, which validate a muscled clean-cut, 90s, international gay look. Chris left the scene voluntarily, his particular niche decimated by the epidemic. The new 90s leather scene in Sydney is now organized by younger, less covert men. Chris might still reside in the centre of inner-Sydney gay life, but he lives beyond even its sexual fringe. Paul is thin, edgy and dresses like a 'Westy', a derogatory term used to describe working-class kids from the western suburbs. He spoke of the put-downs he received at the hands of middle-class, university-educated gays. There are those, it seems, who 'own' gayness, and unintentionally exclude those who cannot identify a Mapplethorpe, do not know who Foucault was, have never visited Castro Street, and don't own a double-album set of *Judy Garland Live at Carnegie Hall*.

Other men spoke of differences between themselves and modern inner-city gays; the latter being too radical, too political and, most often, too young. In spite

of the centrality of gayness to these men's lives and their participation in identi-
fiably gay activities and social networks, each has experienced a marginalization,
an exclusion, a lack of 'fit'.

Issues for Future Social Research

There are important issues here for social research to tackle: if gay community
HIV/AIDS organizations and gay community attachment are crucial to stopping
this epidemic, we need to know more about the production of gay community,
its social dynamics, its processes of sexual inclusion and exclusion. We cannot
ignore the effects of this epidemic on the culture and institutions of those communities. And we cannot ignore the continuing impact of social inequality and
sexual oppression, the distortions they produce, the confusion they create and the
desperation they engender.

HIV/AIDS education can benefit from such an analysis. Recently, we have
asked groups of working-class gay men to evaluate gay community education
materials from Australia and abroad, including the UK. These men almost always
chose the most straightforward pamphlets with immediate and direct messages.
Clear uncluttered artwork, devoid of post-modern metaphor, was chosen over
the 'classy' look of other materials. They bypassed 'art' images, Bruce Weber look-
alikes, the iconography of international gay culture. Most often they chose images
of intimacy between men. They expressed the same delight in erotic images, but
argued that they could not hang them at home, because of family, neighbours and
friends. They did not like pornographic images and representations of esoteric
sexual activity.

This critique should remind educators of the heterogeneity of homosexuality.
It is vital to be alert to the hegemony of inner-urban gay culture on educational
thinking, on representations of gayness invoked as educational strategy. This is
very important as community organizations attempt to move beyond their very
successful campaigns for gay community-identified men to reach other non-gay-
identified, homosexually active men.

These men also remind us of the same issues about social inequality which
have dogged school teachers and educationalists for years: issues about language,
literacy, culture, inclusion and relevancy. I watched a 50-year-old clerk struggle
with a complex visual metaphor in some educational material for half an hour in
one of our sessions. He deserved better; after all he had been organizing the only
gay social club in western Sydney for over six years, almost totally unresourced
by any HIV/AIDS organization.

Dissemination

In addition to policy and evaluation advice to government, we feed our findings
directly to the community sector. The community organizations themselves acknowledge the considerable influence of our work on their educational strategy
and policy development. To achieve this, we have adopted a programme of
dissemination which puts reporting to gay community organizations as our first
priority.

This can be a problem in the publish or perish academy. We suffered at times with grant-awarding bodies and academic critics pointing to a lack of refereed publications during our first three years of work. We have remedied this in the last two years, but would rather our success also be judged on our research reports and technical papers, workshops and seminars, national and international conferences, numerous steering committees and consultancies, directed towards and undertaken with community organizations and health workers. Our community feedback sessions have even been listed as festival events in the Sydney Gay and Lesbian Mardi Gras.

There is a challenge here for researchers. Who constitutes our audience? Do we only inform our peers, other researchers through our traditional and slow publishing rituals, hoping for some sort of trickle-down effect on the epidemic? Social research cannot rely only on academic procedures if it is to be of use. Not only do HIV/AIDS practitioners not read journals of applied psychology, media and cultural studies, and sociology research methods, but most do not read out of their discipline either. We are at a disadvantage compared with our medical colleagues, who often take their elaborate infrastructure and resources for granted. HIV/AIDS-specific journals and international conferences have, on the whole, not provided social science and humanities with the same exposure as medical science. It is imperative that social science make more effort to get findings to those who need them as rapidly as possible, and to do so in language and forms accessible to non-academic perusal and appropriation.

Purpose

The relationship between science and social science is a little like that between 'truck drivers' and 'women truck drivers': we have to be twice as good at what we do to be taken seriously. In the face of epidemiology's failure to comprehend the epidemic's dynamics, public-health officials often seek reassurance from social science, and we most often try to provide this through large-scale, expensive surveys. 'Qualitative' or 'close-focus' work is quite often more useful in offering policy advice than 'quantitative' studies. Surveys of knowledge, attitudes and practices answer some questions, and their descriptive accounts are useful at one level. But more theorized investigations of the social processes, through which the epidemic is experienced, are increasingly important.

There is a challenge here for social researchers to develop 'really useful knowledge', to borrow a term from the nineteenth century British working-class education movements. This does not mean utilitarian research. There are issues and concepts to explore which may not answer an immediate need or serve an immediate purpose. The requirement that social science must be observably and immediately of use is to be resisted. The same is not demanded of medical science. There are social research issues and theoretical work to be done of no immediate impact on the epidemic, but which will make a great deal of difference to our history beyond it. It would be desirable to see more social accountability among all researchers, and for social research to explore issues in ways which take greater advantage of the theoretical and methodological sophistication available in the social sciences and humanities.

Social researchers are centrally placed alongside educators and health workers in stopping this epidemic; although the Nobel Prize will undoubtedly go to those who stop the virus. Nevertheless, it remains our task to explain the epidemic in helpful ways and to assist those affected in their experience of it. It is also our job to challenge the schematic, the jargoned, the simplistic and the stereotypical, to ensure our countries continue to pursue a humane and civilized response to the epidemic.

Acknowledgments

The authors wish to acknowledge the assistance of the Social Aspects of the Prevention of AIDS projects and their research teams at Macquarie University and the AIDS Council of New South Wales; the contribution of the gay and bisexual men who participated in the research reported here; and the financial assistance of the Australian Government through the Commonwealth AIDS Research Grants Committee, the New South Wales Government through its AIDS Bureau, the Macquarie University Research Grants Committee, and the Australian Federation of AIDS Organisations.

Notes

1 Unpublished data from the SAPA Triple S Survey, undertaken in 1991 by the AIDS Research Unit, School of Behavioural Sciences, Macquarie University, Sydney.
2 This original SAPA project (Study A) was a joint undertaking by social researchers from the School of Behavioural Sciences at Macquarie University, the University of Sydney, and the AIDS Council of New South Wales. The SAPA project was established in 1986 and funded by the Commonwealth and New South Wales Departments of Health.
3 D. Altman, Department of Politics, La Trobe University, Melbourne. A project on gay community funded by the Commonwealth AIDS Research Grants Committee in 1989.
4 In the CHAP project we are working largely with Anglo-Australian men who have sex with men; therefore, our analysis leaves out the contribution ethnicity and race make to class dynamics in Australia. For a discussion of early CHAP project findings see Connell *et al.* (1991).

References

BURCHAM, J.L., TINDALL, B., MARMOUR, M., COOPER, D.A., BERRY, G. and PENNY, R. (1989) 'Incidence and Risk Factors for Human Immunodeficiency Virus Seroconversion in a Cohort of Sydney Homosexual Men', *Medical Journal of Australia*, 150, pp. 634–9.

CAMPBELL, I.M., BURGESS, P.M., GOLLER, I.E. and LUCAS, L. (1988) *A Prospective Study of Factors Influencing HIV Infection in Homosexual and Bisexual Men*, Melbourne, University of Melbourne, Department of Psychology.

COMMONWEALTH OF AUSTRALIA (1989) *National NIV/AIDS Strategy: A Policy Discussion Paper*, Canberra, Australian Government Publishing Service.

CONNELL, R.W. and KIPPAX, S. (1990) 'Sexuality in the AIDS Crisis: Patterns of Sexual Practice and Pleasure in a Sample of Australian Gay and Bisexual Men', *Journal of Sex Research*, 27, 2, pp. 167–96.

CONNELL, R.W., CRAWFORD, J., KIPPAX, S., DOWSETT, G.W., BOND, G., BAXTER, D., BERG, R. and WATSON, L. (1988) *Social Aspects of the Prevention of AIDS Study A Report No. 1 — Method and Sample*, Sydney, Macquarie University, School of Behavioural Sciences.

CONNELL, R.W., CRAWFORD, J., KIPPAX, S., DOWSETT, G.W., BAXTER, D., WATSON, L. and BERG, R. (1989) 'Facing the Epidemic: Changes in the Sexual Lives of Gay and Bisexual Men in Australia and Their Implications for AIDS Prevention Strategies', *Social Problems*, 36, 4, pp. 384–402.

CONNELL, R.W., CRAWFORD, J., DOWSETT, G.W., KIPPAX, S., SINNOTT, V., RODDEN, P., BERG, R., BAXTER, D. and WATSON, L. (1990) 'Danger and Context: Unsafe Anal Sexual Practice among Homosexual and Bisexual Men in the AIDS Crisis', *Australian and New Zealand Journal of Sociology*, 26, 2, pp. 187–208.

CONNELL, R.W., DOWSETT, G.W., RODDEN, P., DAVIS, M., WATSON, L. and BAXTER, D. (1991) 'Social Class, Gay Men and AIDS Prevention', *Australian Journal of Public Health*, 15, 3, pp. 178–189.

DOWSETT, G.W. (1990) 'Reaching Men Who Have Sex with Men in Australia: An Overview of AIDS Education, Community Intervention and Community Attachment Strategies', *Australian Journal of Social Issues*, 25, 3, pp. 186–98.

DOWSETT, G.W. (1991) 'Social research on AIDS: Examples from Macquarie University, Sydney', *Venereology*, 4, 1, pp. 38–42.

FRAZER, I.H. MCCAMISH, M., HAY, I. and NORTH, P. (1988) 'Influence of Human Immunodeficiency Virus Antibody Testing on Sexual Behaviour in a "High-risk" Population from a "Low-risk" City', *Medical Journal of Australia*, 149, pp. 365–8.

KIPPAX, S., BOND, G., SINNOTT, V., CRAWFORD, J., DOWSETT, G.W., BAXTER, D., BERG, R., CONNELL, R.W. and WATSON, L. (1989) *Social Aspects of the Prevention of AIDS Study A Report No. 4 — Regional Differences in the Responses of Gay and Bisexual Men to AIDS: The Australian Capital Territory*, Sydney, Macquarie University, School of Behavioural Sciences.

KIPPAX, S., CRAWFORD, J., DOWSETT, E.W., BOND, E., SINNOTT, V., BAXTER, D., BERG, R., CONNELL, R.W. and WATSON, L. (1990) 'Gay Men's Knowledge of HIV Transmission and "Safe" Sex: A Question of Accuracy', *Australian Journal of Social Issues*, 25, 3, pp. 199–219.

NATIONAL CENTRE IN HIV EPIDEMIOLOGY AND CLINICAL RESEARCH (1991) *Australian HIV Surveillance Report, January 1991*, 7, Supplement 1, Sydney, University of New South Wales.

RODDEN, P. (1990) *Social Aspects of the Prevention of AIDS Study A Technical Report No. 9 — HIV Antibody Test Status*, Sydney, Macquarie University, School of Behavioural Sciences.

SOLOMON, P.J. and WILSON, S.R. (1990) 'Projections of Acquired Immune Deficiency Syndrome in Australia', in P.J. SOLOMON, C. FAZEKAS DE ST GROTH and S.R. WILSON (Eds), *Projections of Acquired Immune Deficiency Syndrome in Australia Using Data to the End of September 1989*, National Centre for Epidemiology and Population Health, Working Papers No. 16, 1–10, Canberra, Australian National University.

VADASZ, D. and LIPP, J. (Eds) (1990) *Feeling Our Way: Gay Men Talk about Relationships*, Melbourne, Designer Publications.

2   AIDS, the Media and Health Policy

Virginia Berridge

AIDS, so one policy analyst has argued, may be the 'first media disease' (Street, 1988). But AIDS is by no means the first disease to have a strong media component in its construction and presentation. Historically, disease has long been mediated by its presentation in the press. Cholera, for example, was a key disease in terms of press attention (Morris, 1976). Other diseases killed more widely but few attracted such a range of coverage — from religious periodicals and medical journals, from radical newspapers and magazines on household management; from the educational and temperance press and the literary and scientific papers. The sheer amount of press and periodical focus on the disease helped stimulate a general sense of fear and dread. More recently the media presentation of disease as, for example, in the post-World War I flu epidemic, or the polio epidemic in the 1950s, has been significant in helping structure public responses (Crosby, 1976; Paul, 1971).

AIDS, then, is not the first media disease in the sense of definition in and presentation by the media; but it has had a very high media profile. There is a clear comparison with a disease like hepatitis B. Hepatitis B has many similarities to AIDS — in particular in terms of the main groups affected and routes of transmission. It is also vastly more infectious than HIV. But it has had nothing like the same media attention. One American historian has in fact argued that hepatitis B received scant media coverage there because of the particular threat it posed to health service personnel. Medical experts, the traditional source of information on health and medical matters for the media, were silent on hepatitis B because of the perceived danger of a public and political backlash (Muraskin, 1988).

There were differences in strategies over AIDS. That disease is clearly significant, although not historically unique, in terms of its prominence in the media. But what, conversely, has the significance of the media been in relation to AIDS? This is a potentially vast area for research and analysis, and this chapter discusses two aspects: the relationship of the media to the policy process, both at a governmental level and in terms of the impact of public opinion on policy; and the definition of AIDS as a scientific issue in the media. The overall focus is on the notion of the effect of the media. As Jean Seaton has argued, the idea of a single grand 'media effect' is no longer seen as useful in media studies (Seaton, 1989). 'Media effect' is more a question of differential effects on different groups in society. It may well be, she argues, that the impact of the media on small groups in the elite or in government may be the most important aspect to consider. This chapter sees the relationship of AIDS, the media and health policy within that framework. It argues that most analysis has so far focused almost exclusively on the press 'gay plague' presentation of AIDS. Yet the relationship of the media to the eventual consensual type of policy response appears to have been far more significant.

Current Interpretations of AIDS Policy-making and the Media

Two broad interpretations of AIDS policy-making are currently in play. One, the first to enter the field, analyses AIDS in the context of the New Right predomin- ance of the 1980s and the assertion of Thatcherite values. AIDS, in this sense, has been interpreted as an opportunity for the New Right and for the resurgence of the moral majority, a vehicle for the reassertion of the values of family relationships, of chastity before marriage and fidelity within it; and, most crucially, for the condemnation and isolation of sexual deviance (Watney, 1988; Weeks, 1988). AIDS provided a golden opportunity for moral entrepreneurs to undermine the changes of the 1960s and 1970s. Jeffrey Weeks writes:

> There have been three major strands in the moral and sexual shifts of the past generation: a secularization of moral attitudes, a liberalisation of popular beliefs and behaviours, and a greater readiness to value and re- spect social, cultural and sexual diversity. The significance of the AIDS crisis is that it can be used to call into question each of these, and to advance a justification for a return to that 'normal moral behaviour' which acts as a yardstick by which to measure the supposed decline of moral standards. (Weeks, 1988, pp. 12–13)

This line of thinking emphasizes AIDS as a catalyst for reactionary change. The other broad position on AIDS policy-making, however, emphasizes elements of continuity. It argues that AIDS attracted a great deal of attention; but when the heat had died down and the noise died away, what emerged was 'business as usual', a victory for the liberal biomedical elite and for notions of consensus (both long dominant in this interpretation at least, although the idea of consensus has proved controversial) in post war British policy-making. AIDS was not unusual, or a radical shift in policy-making terms; what was striking was the familiarity of the means used to deal with the issue. AIDS policy-making was a top-down process in which the role of the medical profession was of key importance. Professional and political consensus was the key to policy-making; and AIDS was dealt with according to existing conceptual models (Fox, Day and Klein, 1989; Day and Klein, 1990; Street, 1988).[1]

The role of the media has played some part in both these analyses, but in particular a critique of the press presentation of AIDS has been central to the 'New Right resurgence' approach. It has been argued that the tabloid press presented a view of AIDS as a 'gay plague' which helped reinforce notions of 'moral panic' and of homophobia which were all of a piece with the overall ideological reaction of the decade (Meldrum, 1990). Simon Watney argues:

> After five years of reporting on the AIDS epidemic it is clear that British TV and press coverage is locked into an agenda which blocks out any approach to the subject which does not conform in advance to the values and language of a profoundly homophobic culture — a culture, that is, which does not regard gay men as fully or properly human. . . . (Watney, 1988, p. 52)

The relationship of the media to the establishment of consensual models of policy-making has received some attention (Street, 1988); but the 'gay plague' interpretation has been more prominent.

The Chronology of AIDS Policies 1981–91

In considering the validity of these interpretations, the notion of change over time needs first to be introduced. For policy-making — and the media response to AIDS — has not been static, and responses have not remained the same across the decade. The chronology of policy-making and the related media response must be considered. Policy-making around AIDS can be seen as a sequence of policy stages, with early policy-making input coming from the bottom up — only later to be replaced by a top-down model of policy-making. The different 'policy-making traditions' of distinct areas of policy also need to be remembered.

So far as the chronological framework goes, policy development can be divided into three broad stages (Berridge and Strong, forthcoming; Berridge, forthcoming). From 1981 to 1986 AIDS was an open policy arena. There were no established policy advisory mechanisms, or recognized 'policy community' around the disease. There was the opportunity for policy input 'from below' and from a range of groups outside the normal expert advisory circles. Gay activists, clinicians and scientists from a range of involved areas — immunology, genito-urinary medicine, cancer research — joined in an alliance, sometimes uneasy, with public health interests in the Department of Health. This 'policy community' around the disease was united in its focus on the need for urgent action by government, and the dangers of the heterosexual spread of the disease. This period of policy-making from below was followed in 1986–87 by a relatively short time of what can be called 'national war-time emergency', where AIDS did indeed become a political priority at the highest level. The establishment of the Cabinet committee on AIDS underlined the seriousness with which the government viewed the issue. The 14.5 million pounds given to the MRC's AIDS Directed Programme aiming at the search for a vaccine, the replacement of the Health Education Council by the Health Education Authority with a large AIDS component, also stressed the exceptional nature of the response. But this pitch of reaction was relatively short-lived; from around 1988 it was succeeded by a period of routinization and 'normalization' of the disease. Some of the key protagonists in the early years became less central to policy development. AIDS became a normal part (although with ring fenced funding) of health services. The perception of AIDS as a chronic rather than an epidemic disease established its hegemony; maintenance treatment with AZT and the issue of early treatment of asymptomatic infection contributed to this framework. The problem in policy terms became one of maintaining AIDS salience on the policy agenda.

The Overall Shape of the Media Response

The overall shape of the media (and in particular the press) response appears broadly to have paralleled the chronology of policy development. Four stages can be distinguished: 1981–83, 1983–85, 1986–87 and from 1988 onward. The earliest stage in the early 1980s was the classic period of 'gay plague' presentation in the press. There was relatively little mainstream press coverage; but cases of gay men with AIDS in the United States nevertheless reinforced the idea of AIDS as a disease of others. The terminology of gay plague was used across the press, in quality as well as tabloid papers. Take, for example, *The Sun* in May 1983 with 'Watchdogs in "Gay Plague" Blood Probe'; *The Daily Telegraph* 'Wages of Sin. A Deadly Toll'; *The Sun* again 'US Gay Blood Plague Kills Three in Britain' and in July 1983 the *People* 'What the Gay Plague Did to Handsome Kenny'.[2]

The presentation of these cases and discussion of possible links between disease and the use of nitrites and promiscuous sexual relationships certainly focused on gays as a 'risk group'. It also fitted well within existing parameters of media interest, in particular the long established tradition of sexual sensationalism in the popular press (Berridge, 1978). From mid-1983 the focus within the press shifted to encompass the possibility of heterosexual transmission. Two issues brought this about: questions concerning the safety of the blood supply, and discussion about possible origins in Africa.

It was the blood issue which first crystallized the heterosexual issue in the UK. In May 1983 *The Mail on Sunday* ran a story about hospitals using what it called 'killer blood'.[3] Two men were in hospital in London and Cardiff suspected of having developed AIDS after routine transfusions for haemophilia with imported Factor VIII. In the following year, debates in the medical press about the rival claims of the Haitian and the African connections for AIDS also spilled over into the tabloid and quality presentations (see Chapter 3, this volume). But the theme of 'gay plague' still remained a consistent one. In the British context the particular case which brought press attention to a peak came in the early months of 1985. This was the death of Greg Richards, the chaplain in Chelmsford prison. News reporters were hanging about the prison for a week or two before his death; and press reporting laid emphasis on the possibility of the wider transmission of the virus, either through sexual relationships with prisoners, or via more general routes of contagion. As a result prison officers blocked all movement in or out of the jail. Colin Steel, chairman of the local branch of the Prison Officers' Association, was quoted as saying, 'The mere mention of AIDS strikes sheer terror into people and our members are obviously very worried. The 160 officers at Chelmsford have been instructed not to move any prisoners, nor accept arrivals from other prisons. All we are asking for is clarification of the risks involved.'[4]

The possibility of an 'outbreak' of AIDS at Chelmsford, or in other jails, was widely discussed.[5] This fearful response to the potential for epidemic heterosexual spread via gays — or via other routes — continued throughout 1985 with articles on the threat to the blood supply. This stage of gay plague/heterosexual spread culminated in reporting of the illness and death of Rock Hudson, which dominated AIDS stories in the UK press from July to October 1985. This was a world-wide media event. In other countries the shape of AIDS reporting was broadly similar. An analysis of Australian news stories found a similar early two-stage response punctuated by growing concern about the blood supply (French and Duffin, 1986).

In France a period of panic and fear was represented in the press and also peaked in 1985 (Herzlich and Pierret, 1989).

The media obviously played a key role in the period of national emergency response in Britain, and it was at this stage that the role of television became particularly significant. The routinization and normalization of AIDS in policy terms since 1988 has also been reflected in the shape of media coverage. There was a decline in the intensity of reporting. After the peak of the 1987 media campaign came a reaction against the notion of heterosexual spread. Graham Turner, in an article in *The Sunday Telegraph* in 1988, maintained that heterosexual spread had been propagated by a 'gay conspiracy' with access to government; gay activists had defended their promiscuous lifestyle by deflecting attention to the broader issue.[6] *The Sunday Times* also took up the 'myth of heterosexual spread' from a different angle, claiming that the supposed epidemic was being used as a threat to reassert family values and to deny the young the joys of sexual liberation. AIDS quite often made the news only as part of stories which had a more general sexual component. In 1988 a complaint to the Press Council about *The Mail on Sunday*'s 'alarmist' presentation of a Masters and Johnson sexual survey was rejected because the paper was said to be simply relaying the authors' contribution to the debate on AIDS. Reporting of the cancellation of the national sex survey in 1989 also had a dual focus: on AIDS, but also a more general context of sexual sensationalism which had long been a feature of the British press.[7] The media presentation of AIDS had become normalized. It had also, in the words of one news editor, become a 'boring story. . . . The only stories now would be a miracle cure or a massive rise in heterosexual spread — AIDS is a buried subject.'[8]

The chronology and shape of media attention provided a fairly classic illustration of what Downs has called the 'issue attention cycle', the rise, peak and decline of interest in a policy issue (Downs, 1972). Miller *et al.* (forthcoming) in an analysis of US press coverage found a similar pattern over a slightly different period. The shape of media coverage also conforms to analyses of reporting of other health-related conditions, where the peaks of media coverage have rarely coincided with the height of the 'problem' in quantitative terms. Ives' (1986) analysis of the press coverage of glue sniffing, for example, showed that the peak of coverage occurred well before the rise in numbers of deaths; this, too, was the case with AIDS. The shape of media coverage also indicates that the type of 'gay plague' presentation which has received so much attention in terms of analyses of AIDS reporting was a response which was both historically and media-specific. It was virtually confined to the newspaper press — tabloid and quality — and was particularly prominent in the first two stages of AIDS reporting outlined above.

The 'emergency' and 'normalization' stages of policy development and media coverage have dropped the gay plague angle, but almost at the expense of dropping AIDS and gays coverage altogether. The media focus on heterosexual AIDS has shifted to women as a 'risk group', and women in their traditional role as mothers. The new concern is on the 'threat to the race' via reproduction, and the focus is on women in their child bearing role. Media coverage of World AIDS Day in December 1990 focused specifically on the issue of women and children. Of around 100 AIDS-related stories in *The Sunday Times* between December 1987 and October 1990, only two dealt specifically with gays and AIDS. One of these stories was a piece on the internal problems of the Terrence Higgins Trust. 'Key AIDS Charity in Jeopardy as Bosses Walk Out: Terrence Higgins Trust'.[9]

Deaths of gay men from AIDS were still the bulk of the epidemic (in mid-1989, 95 per cent of people dying of AIDS were gay or bisexual), but media coverage had become 'normalized', along with the policy reaction in general. The appearance of a character with AIDS in a leading TV soap opera, *East Enders*, emphasized this normalization, as did the sympathetic, albeit sensational coverage of the actor Ian Charleson's death in 1990. AIDS had disappeared as a 'gay plague' or, in an alternative formulation, as a gay issue. This shift in media presentation was reinforced by external contributions to the press, in particular in obituaries, a rapidly growing feature of the 1980s quality dailies. An obituary such as that of David E. Thompson in *The Independent* in 1990, 'He was never ashamed that AIDS had called to collect . . .', was a rarity.[10]

The Changing Media Definition of AIDS as a Scientific Issue

The definition and establishment of AIDS as a particular type of scientific issue was also an important aspect of the shape of media coverage of the disease. AIDS was not only an 'open' policy area in its early years, but initially at least an 'open' scientific one as well. The media's role in shaping official and public perceptions of the scientific parameters around AIDS was an important one. Herzlich and Pierret have noted how the French media were important in constructing the disease for society. AIDS as a disease can be seen as in part socially constructed through the media. The advent of AIDS has to some analysts seemed to undermine the social constructionist case in relation to disease (Rosenberg, 1988). Treichler (1988), however, has argued the case for social constructionism more strongly; 'even scientific characterizations of the reality of AIDS are always partly founded upon prior and deeply entrenched cultural narratives. . . . The name AIDS — and indeed the entire biomedical discourse that surrounds it — in part *constructs* the disease and helps make it intelligible.' She points to the establishment of HIV as an exclusive definition, so that other alternatives, for example later claims that HIV does not lead to AIDS, can be dismissed as 'quackery' (Treichler, 1991).

The media have a role to play in legitimating scientific orthodoxies of this kind; this process can be traced in the British media response. The changing shape of scientific definitions and the interaction between different forms of scientific orthodoxy are also important. Particular scientific positions and forms of knowledge have also been historically specific. Biomedical discourse, as in Treichler's analysis, has significantly constructed AIDS as a disease. But there has also been a varying balance of power between AIDS as an epidemiological issue and AIDS as a biomedical one, and the consequences in terms of theories of causation and context; media reporting has both represented and legitimated these orthodoxies. Oppenheimer (1988) has traced the process in the early US response to AIDS whereby epidemiological definitions of the syndrome achieved initial primacy. From 1981 until the isolation of a new virus, epidemiology played a central role in the characterisation of HIV infection. The results were equivocal — with HIV conceptualized, on the one hand, in its social context, on the other, offering a choice of models and hypotheses which were themselves socially constructed and offering opportunities for moral judgment. After the Gallo/Montagnier discovery, the disease was increasingly conceptualized in terms of the infectious agent, the virus. Interest in a multifactorial model diminished. The epidemiological focus appeared, too, in the British press presentation of the issue; the earliest accounts dealt with the epidemiology of the disease and the possible consequences in terms of epidemic spread. Professor Michael Adler of the Middlesex Hospital was reported as saying, at the setting up of a working group of AIDS experts,' . . . people think it is a blood-borne disease which behaves like a virus, but we don't really know what we are looking for. . . . There has been a lot of under-reporting because people have not thought to contact the Communicable Disease Surveillance Centre about their cases.'

The work of the Communicable Disease Surveillance Centre in Colindale and the 'search for numbers' figured largely in the early press presentation of the issue.[11] Reporting the statistics of AIDS was an important part of the early media response. The epidemiological definition of the disease in terms of 'risk groups' also derived from these scientific parameters. The publication of the Gallo/ Montagnier studies in *Science* in May 1984 shifted attention to AIDS as a clinical/ biomedical issue, and the agent host model became dominant. The British press had run stories speculating about a possible viral cause, but the shift in press reporting to a biomedical paradigm came in the latter months of 1984, although, as Wellings (1988) has noted, the identification of a specific pathogen as a cause of AIDS did not eliminate the opportunity to attach blame to selected groups who fell prey to the disease. The biomedical definition of AIDS was important at a policy level. Epidemiological and biomedical definitions continued to interact in particular via the media. The Cox and Day reports in 1988 and 1990, significantly revising the epidemiological predictions downwards, received prominent media coverage and helped in the 'myth of heterosexual spread' press thesis.[12] Conversely, press presentation of epidemiological figures which seemed to indicate the opposite helped raise AIDS policy salience in 1990 and put the issue of heterosexual spread at least temporarily back in the public eye.[13] The news editor's definitions of the newsworthiness of AIDS (quoted above) depended on its scientific constructions, both epidemiological and biomedical.

Some analysts of the media coverage of AIDS, Wellings for example, have seen the presentation of the 'science of AIDS' as a case study of media distortion, in both the biomedical and the epidemiological spheres. Bias there certainly was in various forms: but media presentations should also be seen in a framework which takes account of the interplay between different scientific constructions of disease and their presentation to the public. In that process of presentation an important mediating role has been played by the producers of the media messages. The role of journalists, and in particular of the health and medical correspondents who defined the science of AIDS to a lay audience, needs to be considered. Karpf (1988) has shown how these correspondents rely heavily on 'orthodox' medical sources for stories. This also appears to have been the case for AIDS. Journalists often relied on medical experts for definitions.[14] The former medical correspondent of a quality daily commented that his paper operated a screening system for medical news; nothing on AIDS was covered until it had appeared in the medical press, in particular the *British Medical Journal, Lancet* or *Nature*. Once this type of information had started to come on stream for AIDS, there were doctors who could provide information — 'people you could rely on'.[15] Some journalists, in the UK as in the US, extended their interpretive role further; they published 'instant histories' presenting science and policy to a lay audience (Connor and Kingman, 1988, 1989; McKie, 1986; Shilts, 1987).

The Media and the Policy Process

The media helped to construct AIDS as a scientific issue in the public domain; but they also had an impact on the policy process around AIDS. This section will consider three aspects of that impact: the media's construction of the issue for the gay community; the way in which the 'policy community' around AIDS used the media; and the particular impact of the media in stimulating a high-level political reaction to the disease.

The media were certainly of importance in alerting gays to the dangers of the syndrome. Articles in the gay press, for example the series by Julian Meldrum in *Capital Gay*, 'Meldrum on AIDS', which ran from 1984, fed the changing shape of available knowledge into a vacuum. In spring 1983 a Horizon documentary, 'Killer in the Village', had a particular impact. The London Lesbian and Gay Switchboard opened a special hotline which was inundated after the programme. One gay participant in events commented, 'Many of us were being educated through the media and trying to relate that to oneself.'[16] The media were of importance in helping form a cohesive gay community specifically organized round AIDS (Berridge, forthcoming).

Gays were also part of a wider emergent 'policy community' around AIDS. This community was notable for its media consciousness. 'Media effect' here was not just a top-down process but an interrelationship between policy activists — gays, clinicians and scientists — and the media. All were prepared to use the media to achieve the general policy aims of pressing for urgent action; of stressing the dangers of epidemic spread to the general population; and of pressing a non-punitive response. This media focus was a conscious strategy. Tony Whitehead, then Chair of the Steering Committee of the Terrence Higgins Trust, recalled:

> We had to be seen as a professional body dealing with other professionals, not as a proselytising body. I groomed myself PR wise and pestered professional broadcasters to train me. . . . I didn't have to lose my identity as a gay man. I could wear a suit rather than be festooned with badges. I was the kind of son any mother would want. . . .[17]

The other new 'AIDS experts' — the doctors and scientists — were also prepared to use the media to be openly critical of lack of action. In a more established policy area, internal expert policy advisory mechanisms would have been available, but these did not exist for AIDS until 1985. So experts used the media and entered alliances with gay activists — sometimes uneasy. As one gay man recalled, 'We were always united in front of the cameras — even if we were falling out afterwards.'[18] A bottom-up concept of media effect is, of course, no more monolithic than a top-down one. The relationship here was a symbiotic and sometimes a tense one. The media were not always receptive to the advances of the AIDS policy community. A news editor recalled, 'Charles Farthing became boring. . . . By about 1985–6 I would have turned down a story that had a Charles Farthing line in it. . . . The press are pretty adept at stopping people who are manipulating them . . . they're Rentaquotes. . . .'[19]

The policy community nevertheless stirred up concern over AIDS via the media; and this growing media focus on AIDS, in particular on television, does appear to have helped structure the central government response. The period of high-level government reaction over the disease in late 1986 was preceded by a spate of media presentations on the threat of AIDS, 'Newsnight' and 'Weekend World' among them. It is said that government ministers at the Department of Health were stimulated by these programmes into seeing AIDS as an urgent issue which merited a government response. Certainly the programmes were reacting on a very media-conscious government, one which was sensitive to what was in the press and especially what it saw on television. The media both defined and reinforced issues for politicians too. 'MPs are very slavish to the press . . . they form their judgement on what they read and see on TV. There are all those MPs watching "Newsnight" to see what goes on. There's a strange symbiosis between politics and the media.'[20] It was not only the politicians who were influenced by the media. Civil servants, too, had a close relationship. An article by Peter Jenkins which appeared in *The Sunday Times* on 9 November 1986 and entitled 'The Unappetising Reality of AIDS' was based on a briefing by a very senior government official.

> I never supposed that at one of my occasional lunches with a very senior government official we would be discussing the politics of condoms. Anal sex was mentioned during the avocado, buggery in Her Majesty's prisons as we ate our beef. The very senior official feared 'catastrophe' — nothing had caused him greater loss of sleep in the whole of his long career as a public servant. Nuclear war? 'That might happen if we are all very silly. This is bloody well going to happen — is happening.'[21]

The impact of this piece was later judged as highly significant in determining the government emergency response to AIDS. The particular gatekeeping role of journalists was an important one. Some played a dual role in policy terms. Margaret Jay, for example, moved from media presentation of TV programmes on AIDS ('AIDS — The Last Chance' in October 1986) to subsequent policy activism, via the UK AIDS Foundation (an organization which failed to establish itself because of opposing views over testing), and subsequently as director of the National AIDS Trust, the organization set up in 1987 as mainstream coordinator of the voluntary sector around AIDS.

The Press, Public Opinion and Policy

The media had an impact on government and on particular groups in policy-making circles. But what of the media reaction on more general public attitudes? How far did public opinion enter, if at all, into the policy process; and how far was it structured by the media response? The 'New Right resurgence' interpretations assume that the press stirred up homophobic notions in its readership, and by sensationalist presentation of contradictory evidence, disseminated concepts of contagion and miasma as well as of panic. Some of this analysis derives from earlier work by Cohen and Young on folk devils and the media and uses the concept of the media-induced 'moral panic' (Watney, 1988). There is no doubt that the reaction of some sections of the media did emphasize the idea of contagion, as in the reporting of the Greg Richards case; 'Another Redhot *Sun* Exclusive', on 14 October 1985, concerning a vicar who said he would shoot his son if he had AIDS.

> A vicar vowed yesterday that he would take his teenage son to a moun-
> tain and shoot him if the boy had the deadly disease AIDS. And to make
> his point, the Rev. Robert Simpson climbed a hill behind his church and
> aimed a shotgun at his 18-year-old son Chris. Mr Simpson, 64, said 'Chris
> would not get closer to me than six yards. He would be a dead man.'

It is easy to interpret this type of reporting within a framework of press
distortion and 'moral panic'. But other questions also need to be considered: the
nature of media effect; the constitution and relationship with lay beliefs about disease; and the impact of the press and public opinion on the policy response to AIDS.

So far as media effect goes, there has been criticism recently of the older view
of reinforcement not change, the idea that the press could only reinforce existing
views and could not change them. Research which has focused primarily on
voting behaviour has stressed that, as ties of class and community have loosened
in the 1980s, the media may have a more autonomous relation to belief and
attitudes (Harrop, 1987). The media do structure responses, at least insofar as
voting is concerned; but the impact is a differential one mediated differently within
families and between sexes. Such revisionist views of effect may not be entirely
applicable to non-voting beliefs and attitudes; and certainly a 'top-down' notion
of media effect must also be set in relation to popular beliefs about disease which
have a very long history.

Beliefs about contagion and miasma in relation to disease are long established;
and views of moral responsibility for disease pre-date AIDS. As Rosenberg (1990)
has pointed out, they are one way in which historically populations affected by
epidemics have tried to make sense of them, a way of imposing order on apparent
randomness and chaos. There is no doubt of the extent of public disquiet about
the implications of AIDS at a specific historic conjuncture. The forgetfulness as
well as the 'condescension of posterity' can overlook the undercurrent of rumour
and panic which took hold, especially between 1984 and 1985. 'We were planning
for virtually the whole of the Westminster Hospital to be given over to AIDS
cases', recalled one consultant.[22] 'We thought about a third of the population of
Kensington and Chelsea was going to have AIDS in a few years' time', commented the ex-Director of Social Services (to laughter) at a conference in 1990.[23]

Public opinion and other market research surveys demonstrated a strong
current of opinion in favour of compulsory public health measures such as
quarantine, notification and the compulsory identification of seropositives.[24] Lay
beliefs about contagion in relation to the disease were also widespread (Warwick,
Aggleton and Homans, 1988). 'Moral panic' theory presupposes a top-down media
effect and arises from a view which stresses the media as an agent for producing
the compliance of the masses, a concept which has begun to be critically analyzed
by historians of the press (Hiley, 1991). It would perhaps be more realistic to
analyze a symbiotic relationship where popular views of disease were to some
degree mediated — and reinforced — by the press.

The Role of Television

Ultimately, both the tabloid press and public opinion were ineffective in policy
terms. The furore over 'gay plague' representations has tended to overlook their

complete lack of policy impact. The official consensus formed around 'safe sex' and 'harm minimization', not around quarantine or anti-gay propaganda. The role of television should be considered here. The press presentation of AIDS differed from that of television; these different sections of the media appear to have had a differential impact on the policy process. The press perception, in particular the tabloid view, was closer to the New Right rhetoric of government. But it established no policy credibility; the liberal consensual model advanced on television won. The mounting of AIDS week on television is February 1987 demonstrated television's reinforcement and establishment of consensus. AIDS week was an 'unprecedented peacetime event', the only time since World War II, apart from Apollo moon landings and various Royal weddings, when there had been such cooperation between the two broadcasting companies — and in this case a government department, the DHSS (Alcorn, 1989). The original suggestion, following discussions instigated by Sir Kenneth Stowe, Permanent Secretary at the DHSS, had been for a single programme broadcast simultaneously across all four channels. But it was felt within the Department that television also had to provide information, and in mid-November 1986 a joint DHSS/Cabinet office/BBC meeting decided on the need for the widest possible campaign. By January, joint BBC/TV/DHSS meetings had decided that AIDS week would be at the end of February after the advertising campaign and after Norman Fowler's return from San Francisco, a visit which received extensive news coverage as part of the government and television's public health campaigns.

There was concern throughout the planning of these programmes, and afterwards, about what this cooperation would mean for government control of broadcasting in Britain. This was, for the BBC, a period of intense government pressure. The Peacock Committee had been discussing the question of advertising; Alastair Milne had been sacked as Director General in 1986; and the planned revision of the Obscene Publications Act aimed to extend its provisions to cover television. One broadcaster involved in the planning of AIDS week commented, 'People were beginning to ask — what next? Broadcasters had more or less given up editorial rights . . . and were acting as a government mouthpiece. . . . It made broadcasters reflect on the dangers of giving up editorial freedom and control. . . .'[25] Thus far, then, the use of television fitted into the 'New Right resurgence' interpretation of government control; but at another level it did not. For what emerged on television was not the Right agenda of testing and quarantine, but a victory for the liberal line. AIDS was seen as a threat to the general population, and the message was one of harm minimization, not of morality.

It could not be claimed that television coverage was responsible for this liberal response. Any explanation of that response must raise broader issues of the continuity of pre-Thatcherite political traditions, the reality of the supposed 'Thatcher revolution' in government, and the nature of the consensual response to AIDS. Certainly television, as a more liberal consensual medium than the press, naturally conveyed that range of AIDS coverage. Alcorn (1989) has analyzed one particular programme which went out during AIDS week — the 'AIDS Debate', a special edition of the BCC1 programme, 'Day to Day', which attracted a late-night audience of four and a half million on Friday, 27 February 1987 (Alcorn, 1989). The programme was notable for a clash between the 'New Right' representatives — Christopher Monckton, a past member of Mrs Thatcher's Policy Unit, and Graham Webster-Gardiner of Conservative Family Campaign, both of whom argued for compulsory measures. They were opposed by Michael Adler, arguing on the basis of rights, rather than of practicalities, and by Terry Madeley, a 'photogenic and telegenic' gay man with AIDS, who went on to become something of a television personality during the rest of his life. But the programme's general thrust, despite the appearance of New Right views, was towards the liberal consensus over AIDS, an approach which was reinforced by Robert Kilroy-Silk, the programme's presenter who allied himself openly with the liberal line.

Television reinforced the consensual approach; in doing so, it continued a long established pattern in the relationship of broadcasting to politics. Scannell and Cardiff have defined this historically as the struggle over whether a public service institution like the BBC should act or speak in the national interest or in the public interest (concepts which are often conflated by government). The BBC espoused the 'national interest' at two crucial junctures, the General Strike and the Munich crisis. The BBC was the servant of a 'national community whose general interests it had to express' (Scannell and Cardiff, 1991). Behind that policy lay a concept of society positing a very wide consensus, a dedication to common goals and a lack of social tensions. This type of outlook continued into the 1980s. Public broadcasting again adopted the 'national' rather than the 'public' stance. AIDS week and the role of television coverage of AIDS can thus be seen as exemplifying a long-standing tendency in British public broadcasting; the 'national community'/general population response fitted its existing relationship to politics.

Conclusion

Many aspects of the media's relationship with AIDS remain to be analyzed. The media have, as argued here, affected the policy process around the disease. But AIDS has also had an impact on the pre-existing 'politics of the media'. Take the continuing Murdoch/Maxwell battles, in this case exemplified by *The Sunday Times'* attacks on Robert Maxwell's involvement in the launch of the National AIDS Trust, and Maxwell's subsequent recourse to the Press Council.[26] The continuing role of mass media compaigns around AIDS also deserves analysis (Rhodes and Shaughnessy, 1990). But the focus of this paper has been on media effect on the policy process.

Three broad views of media effect can be distinguished, all deriving from different, and often historic, schools of media analysis (Seaton and Pimlott, 1987). The 'liberal traditionalist' view saw the media as the 'Fourth Estate', as a check on the powerful. In the inter-war period the Frankfurt School, among others, saw the media as, by contrast, the servant of the powerful, as a means of producing the compliance of the masses. Another view sees the media as implicated in the political process, as a means whereby different interests are expressed. Many analyses of AIDS and the media have adopted the 'social control' approach, based on the Frankfurt position. The third model is also applicable to the relationship between the media and AIDS policy-making. The role of the media has been important, but not monolithic, and there have been clear differences between the press, on the one hand, and television, on the other. In policy terms, television was more important. As itself a liberal consensual medium, long allied to the concept of a 'national' rather than a 'public community', it was a key medium for reinforcing the consensual reaction to AIDS at the policy level.

Notes

1 Street (forthcoming) has also noted that different areas of policy-making had different policy traditions. For example, decision-making in terms of treatment policies was much more localized than in a 'political' area such as health education.

2 These headlines come from *The Sun*, 2 May 1983; *The Daily Telegraph*, 2 May 1983; *The Sun*, 8 May 1983; *The People*, 24 July 1983.

3 *Mail on Sunday*, 1 May 1983.

4 *The Daily Telegraph*, 6 February 1985.

5 *The Star*, 15 February 1985.

6 *The Sunday Telegraph*, 5 June 1988.

7 *Mail on Sunday*, 24 July 1988.

8 Interview, news editor, October 1989.

9 *The Sunday Times*, 29 May 1988.

10 *Independent*, 27 July 1990; A *Guardian* correspondent (15 January 1990) pointed to the failure to mention AIDS as a cause of death in obituaries. Geoffrey Wheatcroft discussed this issue in the *Independent Magazine*, 26 May 1990, arguing that UK obituaries were less open than US ones; and any disease to which social stigma attached was rarely mentioned in obituaries.

11 See, for example, 'Prevalence of AIDS in UK Underestimated', an article in *Medical News*, 28 April 1983, drawing on a *Lancet* piece of 16 April 1983. A. Scott (1987) 'AIDS and the Experts', *New Scientist*, 5 March discusses the changing scientific definitions of AIDS and their media presentation albeit in a Whiggish 'march of scientific knowledge' framework.

12 See digest of press coverage in 'Normal Sex', *AIDS Newsletter*, 4, 17, 1989, pp. 2–3.

13 The work of the All Party Parliamentary Group on AIDS and its press conference on the latest figures in 1990 were important in establishing this as an epidemiological issue.

14 See, for example, a profile of Sir (then Doctor) Donald Acheson by Thompson Prentice in *The Times*, 7 November 1985, which relays the views of its subject without further analysis.

15 Interview, former medical correspondent, March 1991.

16 Interview, gay community worker, April 1990.

17 Interview, Tony Whitehead, July 1989.

18 Comment from gay writer, July 1989.

19 Interview, news editor, October 1989.

20 Interview, news editor, October 1989.

21 Peter Jenkins, 'The Unappetising Reality of AIDS', *The Sunday Times*, 9 November 1986.

22 Interview, cardiologist, April 1991.

23 Talk by Andrew Henderson at conference on AIDS and the local authority response, September 1990.

24 Christopher Monckton, deputy editor of *Today* and a former member of Mrs Thatcher's Policy Unit, presented the results of an opinion poll in favour of the compulsory identification of seropositives on 'The AIDS Debate' on television in February 1987. See K. Alcorn (1989) 'AIDS in the Public Sphere', in E. Carter, and S. Watney (Eds), *Taking Liberties: AIDS and Cultural Politics*, London, Serpent's Tail.

25 Interview, media worker, January, 1989.

26 See, for example, *The Sunday Times*, 20 December 1987, 'Maxwell in New Row on AIDS Charity'; 7 February 1988, 'Maxwell Pays Up'. Two of the 'quality'

Sundays, *The Sunday Times* and *The Observer*, have both run campaigns round an 'innocent victims' theme, haemophiliacs with AIDS in *The Sunday Times* and those given infected blood via transfusion in *The Observer*.

References

ALCORN, K. (1989) 'AIDS in the Public Sphere', in E. CARTER and S. WATNEY (Eds), *Taking Liberties: AIDS and Cultural Politics*, London, Serpent's Tail.

BERRIDGE, V. (1978) 'Popular Sunday Papers and Mid-Victorian Society', in G. BOYCE, J. CURRAN and P. WINGATE (Eds), *Newspaper History: From the Seventeenth Century to the Present Day*, London, Constable.

BERRIDGE, V. (forthcoming) 'The Early Years of AIDS in the UK, 1981–6 an Historical Perspective', in P. SLACK and T. RANGER (Eds), *Epidemics and Ideas*, Oxford, Oxford University Press.

BERRIDGE, V. and STRONG, P. (forthcoming) 'AIDS in the UK: Contemporary History and the Study of Policy', *Twentieth Century British History*.

CONNOR, S. and KINGMAN, S. (1988, 1989) *The Search for the Virus*, Harmondsworth, Penguin Books.

CROSBY, A. (1976) *Epidemic and Peace 1918*, Westport, Conn., Greenwood Press.

DAY, P. and KLEIN, R. (1990) 'Interpreting the Unexpected: The Case of AIDS Policy Making in Britain', *Journal of Public Policy*, 9, pp. 337–53.

DOWNS, A. (1972) 'Up and Down with Ecology: The Issue Attention Cycle', *Public Interest*, 28, pp. 38–50.

FOX, D.M., DAY, P. and KLEIN, R. (1989) 'The Power of Professionalism: AIDS in Britain, Sweden and the United States', *Daedalus*, 118, pp. 93–112.

FRENCH, R. and DUFFIN, R. (1986) *'Mossies Could Spread AIDS': Australian Media References on AIDS, 1981–1985*, Sydney, Gay History Project.

HARROP, M. (1987) 'Voters', in J. SEATON and B. PIMLOTT (Eds), *The Media in British Politics*, Aldershot, Gower/Avebury.

HERZLICH, C. and PIERRET, J. (1989) 'The Construction of a Social Phenomenon: AIDS in the French Press', *Social Science and Medicine*, 29, 11, pp. 1235–42.

HILEY, N. (1991) 'News, Propaganda and Popular Culture in Britain', Paper given at the Social History Society Conference, Lincoln.

IVES, R. (1986) 'The Rise and Fall of the Solvents Panic', *Druglink*, 1, 4, pp. 10–12.

KARPF, A. (1988) *Doctoring the Media: The Reporting of Health and Medicine*, London, Routledge.

MCKIE, R. (1986) *Panic: The Story of AIDS*, Wellinborough, Thorsons.

MELDRUM, J. (1990) 'The Role of the Media and the Reporting of AIDS', in B. ALMOND (Ed.), *AIDS: A Moral Issue*, London, Macmillan.

MILLER, J., et al. (forthcoming) 'Changing Levels of Public Interest of AIDS in the 1980s', Unpublished paper.

MORRIS, R.J. (1976) *Cholera 1832: The Social Response to an Epidemic*, London, Croom Helm.

MURASKIN, W. (1988) 'The Silent Epidemic: The Social, Ethical and Medical Problems Surrounding the Fight against Hepatitis B', *Journal of Social History*, 22, pp. 277–98.

OPPENHEIMER, G. (1988) 'In the Eye of the Storm: The Epidemiological Construction of AIDS', in E. FEE and D.M. FOX (Eds), *AIDS: The Burdens of History*, Berkeley, Calif., University of California Press.

PAUL, J.R. (1971) *A History of Poliomyelitis*, New Haven, Conn., Yale University Press.

RHODES, T. and SHAUGHNESSY, R. (1990) 'Compulsory Screening: Advertising AIDS in Britain, 1986–89', *Policy and Politics* 18, 1, pp. 55–61.

ROSENBERG, C. (1988) 'Disease and Social Order in America: Perceptions and Expectations', in E. FEE and D.M. FOX (Eds), *AIDS: The Burdens of History*, Berkeley, Calif., University of California Press.

ROSENBERG, C. (1990) 'What is an Epidemic?' in S.R. GRAUBARD (Ed.), *Living with AIDS*, Cambridge, Mass., MIT Press.

SCANNELL, P. and CARDIFF, D. (1991) *A Social History of Broadcasting. Vol. 1 I 1922–1939: Serving the Nation*, Oxford, Blackwell.

SEATON, J. (1989) 'Bias and Power in the Media', *Contemporary Record*, 2, 5, pp. 8–11.

SEATON, J. and PIMLOTT, B. (1987) 'Introduction', in J. SEATON and B. PIMLOTT (Eds), *The Media in British Politics*, Aldershot, Gower/Avebury.

SHILTS, R. (1987) *And the Band Played On: Politics, People and the AIDS Epidemic*, Harmondsworth, Penguin Books.

STREET, J. (1988) 'British Government Policy on AIDS', *Parliamentary Affairs*, 41, pp. 490–508.

STREET, J. (forthcoming) 'AIDS Policies in the UK', Paper prepared for nine nation comparative study of AIDS policies.

TREICHLER, P. (1988) 'AIDS, Gender and Biomedical Discourse: Current Contests for Meaning', in E. FEE and D.M. FOX (Eds) *AIDS: The Burdens of History*, Berkeley, Calif., University of California Press.

TREICHLER, P. (1991) 'AIDS, HIV and the Cultural Construction of Reality', in G. HERDT and S. LINDENBAUM (Eds), *The Social Sciences in the Age of AIDS*, London, Sage.

WATNEY, S. (1988) 'AIDS, "Moral Panic" Theory and Homophobia', in P. AGGLETON and H. HOMANS (Eds), *Social Aspects of AIDS*, Lewes, Falmer Press.

WARWICK, I., AGGLETON, P. and HOMANS, H. (1988) 'Young Peoples' Health Beliefs and AIDS', in P. AGGLETON and H. HOMANS (Eds), *Social Aspects of AIDS*, Lewes, Falmer Press.

WEBSTER, C. (1990) 'Conflict and Consensus: Explaining the British Health Service', *Twentieth Century British History*, 1, 2, pp. 115–51.

WEEKS, J. (1988) 'Love in a Cold Climate', in P. AGGLETON and H. HOMANS (Eds), *Social Aspects of AIDS*, Lewes, Falmer Press.

WELLINGS, K. (1988) 'Perceptions of Risk-Media Treatments of AIDS', in P. AGGLETON and H. HOMANS (Eds), *Social Aspects of AIDS*, Lewes, Falmer Press.

3 'African AIDS': The Media and Audience Beliefs

Jenny Kitzinger and David Miller

> If we relinquish the compulsion to separate true representations of AIDS from false ones and concentrate instead on the process and consequences of representation and discursive production, we can begin to sort out how particular versions of truth are produced and sustained, and what cultural work they do in given contexts. Such an approach . . . raises questions not so much about truth as about power and representation. (Treichler, 1989, p. 48)

The prevalence of HIV infection in Africa and the question of the origins of HIV are contentious and much debated topics. The scientific validity of the African origin theory has been called into question, and the 'Green Monkey Theory' (the idea that HIV originated among African monkeys and then spread to human beings) has now been rejected by some of the scientists who first propounded it (Chirimuuta and Chirimuuta, 1989). The prevalence of infection in different African countries is also not a straightforward matter. For example, the early HIV antibody test cross-reacted with the antibodies to malarial plasmodium, 'resulting in a huge number of false positive results' (Patton, 1990, p. 26). Black scientists, activists, grassroots workers and researchers have challenged the assumptions of much Western scientific theorizing about the origins of HIV, and analysts of the media have highlighted racist subtexts in reporting about AIDS and Africa (see Adams, 1989: Chirimuuta and Chirimuuta, 1989; Critical Health, 1988; Patton, 1990; Sabatier, 1988; Watney, 1988).

However, there is little empirical research exploring how media reporting might actually relate to audience understandings. This chapter focuses on audiences and the role of the media in changing, reinforcing or contributing to ideas about AIDS, Africa and race. It does not argue that HIV either does, or does not, originate in Africa, nor does it seek to deny the terrible suffering caused by HIV in certain parts of Africa. Here we are not directly addressing questions about where the virus 'really' came from or the actual distribution of infection. Instead we are focusing on how different answers to these questions are produced, framed and sustained, what these tell us about the construction of 'AIDS' and 'Africa', and what socio-political consequences they carry with them. This chapter addresses questions such as:

What are people's sources of information about AIDS and Africa?

How is media coverage of AIDS in Africa understood by different audiences?

Why do some people accept and others reject the Africa/AIDS association?

How are audience understandings mediated by structural position, personal experience, political culture and access to alternative versions of reality?

Our aims are to document the distinct nature of media reports about AIDS in Africa, and to demonstrate how many research participants in our work recalled and reconstructed media statements about 'African AIDS'. We argue that such vivid recall is not simply due to the direct influence of media AIDS reporting but is partly dependent on widespread pre-existing ideas about Africa; it is easy for white people in Britain to believe that Africa is a reservoir of HIV infection because 'it fits'.

Methods

The findings presented here are part of the AIDS Media Research Project, an investigation funded by the Economic and Social Research Council into the production, content and audience understandings of HIV/AIDS media messages.[1] The chapter draws on two sorts of analysis: an examination of main news bulletins between 1 October 1986 and 30 April 1990, and in-depth group discussions with fifty-two different audience groups.[2]

It focuses on television news bulletins because, unlike the press, television news is legally supposed to adhere to 'objective' or 'unbiased' standards of reporting. In addition, according to a number of surveys, people consistently cite television as their most important source of information on AIDS (36 per cent), followed by newspapers (31 per cent) (McQueen *et al.*, 1989).

The project team chose to work with discussion *groups* rather than to conduct individual interviews because the aim was to explore how social interaction and identity affect people's understandings. For this reason it was also decided to work with pre-existing groups of people who already lived, worked or socialized together.

Because of an interest in exploring the *diversity* of audience understandings, some groups were chosen because they might be expected to have particular knowledge of, or perspectives on, HIV/AIDS. Others were chosen because, as a group, they were not necessarily expected to have any special interest in this issue. The aim also was to include participants with a range of demographic characteristics. Some groups were specifically selected to ensure that the sample included old people as well as young, English people as well as Scottish, and black people as well as white. Research sessions were conducted with groups as varied as doctors employed in the same infectious diseases unit, male workers on a gay helpline, African journalists, prisoners, school children, office cleaners, members of a retirement group in Kent and a group of women living on the same Glasgow estate (see Figure 3.1).[3]

Each research session lasted about two hours and, in addition to open discussions, research participants were asked individually to complete questionnaires

Figure 3.1   Groups Involved in the Study

I Groups with some occupational interest, involvement or responsibility

Group	Number of groups of this type	Total number of participants in these groups
Doctors	1	4
Nurses/Health visitors	1	6
Social workers	1	4
Drug workers	1	5
NACRO workers[1]	1	3
Police staff	2	16
Prison staff	5	32
Teachers	1	5
African journalists	1	4
Community council workers	1	3

II Groups perceived as 'high risk' or with some special knowledge of, or political involvement in, the issue

Male prostitutes	2	6
Gay men	2	9
Lesbians	2	6
Family of a gay man	1	4
Prisoners	5	28
Clients of NACRO and SACRO[2]	4	27
Clients of drug rehabilitation centre	1	7
Young people in intermediate treatment	1	5

III Groups with no obvious special interest or involvement in the issue

Retired people	3	25
Neighbours	1	4
School students	3	26
Women with children attending playgroup	2	14
Engineers	2	18
Round table group	1	14
American students	1	25
Janitors	1	7
Market researchers	1	3
Cleaners	1	4
College students	3	37
Total number of all groups	52	
Total number of participants in all groups		351

Notes: 1. NACRO — National Association for the Care and Resettlement of Offenders;
2. SACRO — Scottish Association for the Care and Resettlement of Offenders

and collectively to write their own news bulletin using a set of thirteen photographs. The photographs were stills taken from television news and documentary coverage of HIV/AIDS and were chosen to reflect recurring themes and visual images in the media coverage of this topic (see Kitzinger, 1990, for more details

Figure 3.2   The Photograph Which Generated Discussion about 'Africa'

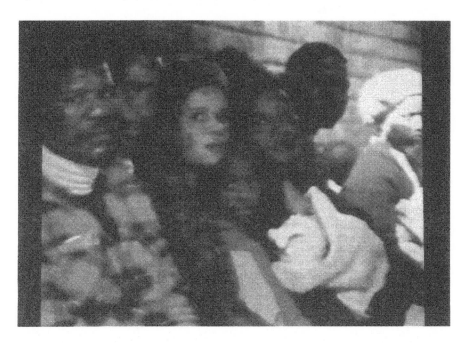

of the methodology). The set of photographs included a picture of a crowd in the street, a laboratory worker looking down a microscope, a government official, a representative from the Terrence Higgins Trust, a doctor, a woman holding a child, a person looking ill in bed, as well as the photograph in Figure 3.2.

Data directly relevant to this chapter were primarily triggered by (i) this photograph, (ii) questions in a questionnaire asking about the prevalence of AIDS in different parts of the world and (iii) debate about where HIV 'came from'.

Results and Discussion

Audience Belief: The Power of the Media

Among our research participants the most popular belief about the origins of HIV was that it came from Africa. Not only was Africa most likely to be identified as the source of HIV but it was also most likely to be identified as having a particularly high prevalence of AIDS. Of the 258 respondents who identified any part of the world as having a particularly high number of reported cases of AIDS, 128 named 'Africa', 28 specified a particular country in, or an area of, Africa and 37 referred to 'the Third World' or the 'underdeveloped world'. According to them, their primary source of information for this belief was the media, in the form of television, newspaper or radio reports (for a detailed presentation of these figures, see Kitzinger and Miller, 1991).[4]

In addition to claiming that the media were their source of information, many participants specifically recalled the ways in which early reporting of AIDS linked it to Africa, Haiti or the Third World.[5] For many people, this sort of reporting was their first encounter with 'the AIDS story'. Asked when he first heard about AIDS, a respondent in the prison sample replied:

> *Resp. 1:* It was when I was reading it in the paper round about '84
> *Int.:* What roughly did it say? What did it convey?
> *Resp. 1:* Something about Africa and AIDS.
>
> (Prisoner, Group 2)

Another man (a member of a 'family' group) commented,

> The first time I ever heard anything about AIDS . . . was in an article about San Francisco . . . and about how Haiti had something to do with it. People from Haiti seemed to be particularly prone to it and that in some way was linked with Africa. (Family group)

Other research participants made statements such as:

> I've just got this idea that AIDS is quite rife over in Africa. I've seen stories about businessmen going across and coming back from Africa with HIV. There have been media stories about it starting in Africa as well. (Lesbian, Group 1)

> The first of it I heard had come from Haiti, and they say that over there there's somewhere in the region of about nearly 80 per cent have got the virus. (Retired person, Group 1)

> I remember in the early days of the campaign them constantly saying that the Haitian community had been one of the first in America, they were always mentioned as one of the high-risk groups. (Market researchers)

The identification of AIDS as a disease of the '4 Hs' had particularly stuck in some people's minds, and the alliteration clearly served as a cue to memory. A gay man said:

> From what I remember is that they talked about three H's there were Haitians involved, it was rife in the Haitians community, and haemophiliacs and heroin users, it must have been the four Hs with homosexuals, and they thought that poppers might play a role. I remember *that* from the programme. [laughter] (Gay man, Group 1)

A doctor commented:

> *Resp. 1:* And everyone could remember the four Hs.
> *Int.:* Which are?
> *Resp. 1:* Homosexuals, heroin addicts, Haitians and haemophiliacs.

At which point his colleague interjected:

> *Resp. 2*:   Haitians . . . that's it. I remember now.
>
> (Doctors)

In addition, participants often recalled detailed accounts of how the virus got from 'over there' to 'here' and were able to reconstruct media statements about 'African AIDS' which echoed media language, concepts and explanatory frameworks, and reiterated statistics, images and even presentational techniques from the television news. This will be illustrated by having a closer look at four themes and highlighting the problems in both the original media presentations and the audience reiteration of the constructs they work with.

'African AIDS': The Construction of a Single 'Africa'

First, we examine the tendency among many research participants to view the African continent as a single, undifferentiated socio-cultural block. As critics, such as Patton (1990) and Watney (1988), have pointed out, the media often present Africa as a homogeneous whole. This is certainly true of much of the three and a half years of television news reports examined. In these reports individual African countries *were* identified but usually only as examples of Africa in general.

In 1987 ITN broadcast a series of reports on what it called 'AIDS in Africa'. Some of the reports were introduced against the background of the graphic shown in Figure 3.3, with comments such as: 'The second of our special series "AIDS in Africa" reports now on Uganda' (ITN 1745, 6 May 1987).

Statistics were then given of HIV infection for the whole of Africa, and a map of Africa was shown with the word 'AIDS' branded across the entire continent and stamped with the words '3 Million Sufferers' (see Figures 3.4 and 3.5).

In the three and a half years of main news bulletins that were examined, the only country to be distinguished as different from the general picture was South Africa. In fact, on one occasion South Africa was described as 'holding the line' against an HIV invasion apparently threatening to surge across the border from black Africa (ITN 2200, 5 December 1986). This crude homogenization of 'black Africa' is reflected in audience statements. Of the 178 people who named the continent of 'Africa' or who talked about 'the Third World' as a place with a high prevalence of AIDS, only twenty-eight felt it necessary (or were able) to be more specific. Parts of the media and many members of the audience groups are ignoring the specific characteristics of AIDS epidemics in different African Countries. As Patton writes: 'Much political and social violence is accomplished by collapsing the many cultures of the African continent in the invention "Africa"' (Patton, 1990, p. 25). The distinctive treatment of South Africa in some television coverage might appear to run counter to Patton's argument, but in fact demonstrates that television news distinctions are often not about territorial boundaries but are based on the difference between black and white.

AIDS as a Black Syndrome

Although there is a paucity of images of black people in the media in general, and perhaps in health education coverage in particular, the media often use images of

Figure 3.3   AIDS in Africa Graphic, ITN, 1987

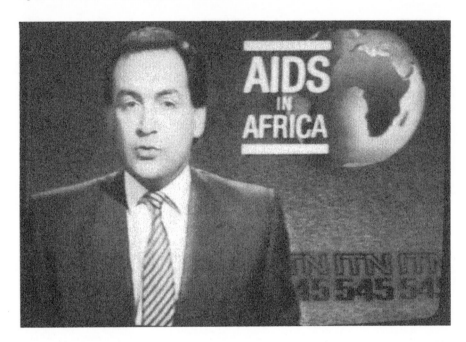

Figure 3.4   'AIDS in Africa': Now 75 Million May Die (ITN 2200, 5 May 1987)

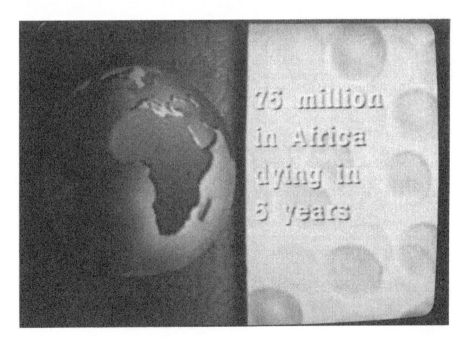

Figure 3.5 In Africa There Are Already an Estimated 3 Million Sufferers with Number of Victims Doubling Every 6 Months (ITN 2200, 2 January 1990)

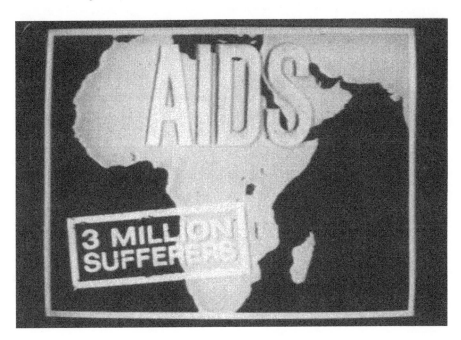

black Africans with AIDS in their reports.[6] Most dramatically, ITN's 1986 end-of-year review used the face of a black man from the Congo to illustrate what the newscaster called 'the face of AIDS' (ITN *Review of the Year*, 30 December 1986; see Figure 3.6). Such associations were also evident in the minds of those research participants who declared that AIDS was common in 'black countries' (Prison staff, Group 2), 'black provinces' (Police staff) and 'black cities' (American student), as well as among 'the ethnic community' (Janitor). Thus the advice from one ex-prisoner that the way to protect yourself from HIV was 'Don't go near the darkies' (SACRO clients).

The Proportion of People Infected

The powerful impression made by images is not surprising in view of other media research (e.g., Philo, 1990). More unusually, however, participants could reproduce statistics about the proportion of infected people in Africa, even if they sometimes confused HIV with AIDS or occasionally exaggerated the figures beyond the range of most media statements. For example, one janitor proclaimed: 'Uganda's hoachin with it. . . . Half the people in Uganda have got AIDS.' Figure 3.7 provides an example of audience and media statements about prevalence of infection in Africa. The statistics given by the media (and the audience) vary wildly. TV news reporters do not even seem to be able to make up their minds about how many people have HIV and AIDS in particular African countries. In

Figure 3.6   The Face of AIDS (ITN 'Review of the Year', 20 December 1986)

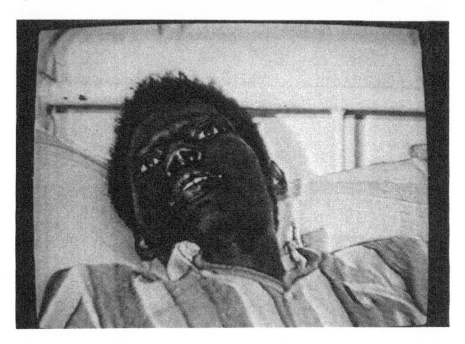

April 1987, for example, the BBC reported that, in Uganda, 'one in every ten people has AIDS' (BBC1 2100, 30 April 1987). Yet by 1990 ITN was reporting, without commenting on previous statements, that HIV infection was apparently much lower. In Uganda, they said, 'one person in sixteen has the virus' (ITN 2200, 2 January 1990).

Such cavalier use of cataclysmic scenarios about the level of infection in Africa partly reflects early errors in antibody testing in Africa where false positive results were picked up from the test's reaction to malarial plasmodium. It also reflects a cavalier approach to African disasters in general where journalists can report: 'A million people may die or maybe two million, we just don't know' (Channel Four News 1900, 2 February 1987). This in turn fits into the view of Africa as a disaster-ridden continent and allows scientists to justify using Africa as a testing ground for drugs, as well as permitting the 'African tragedy' to be used as a dire warning of what could happen 'over here'.

Some audience groups constructed news reports which employed 'the African tragedy' as an example to illustrate some other point rather than focusing on Africa in its own right. In so doing, they sometimes used presentation techniques identical to those used on the news.

News Presentation Techniques

Death in Africa is routinely treated as 'a fact of life'. AIDS in Africa slips neatly into this formula, and in some ways is not even newsworthy in its own right. This was

Figure 3.7 Audience and Media Statements about Prevalence of Infection in Africa

Statement from audience newsgame reports	Statements from actual TV news bulletins
'1 in 3 they say have got the virus' (Clients in drug rehabilitation centre)	'In Lusaka, researchers say one in three men between the ages of thirty and thirty five carries the virus . . .' (C4 News 1900, 2 February 1987)
'Good Evening this is the 6 O'clock News and I'm' Trevor McDonald. . . . In a recent survey done in the Third World, it was found out that over one million people have been infected in the past five years'. (Drug worker)	'Africa already has an estimated 3 million sufferers. In Uganda alone there are around 1 million. One in every sixteen people.' (ITN 1740, 2 January 1990)
'There have been other documentaries where they say that 30 per cent of the prostitutes in Nairobi have it.' (Teachers)	'In Africa a million people could die of AIDS in the next decade or maybe two million, we just don't know.' (C4 News 1900, 2 February 1987)
'30 per cent in Zambia are going to be dead in 5 years.' (Teachers)	'In Africa it is estimated there are 50,000 people with AIDS, twice as many as the rest of the world.' (C4 News 1900, 2 February 1987)
'In East Africa where the problem of HIV infection is now endemic with between 10 per cent and 20 per cent of population affected.' (Doctors)	'Among the adult population AIDS could become the biggest killer within 5 years. According to the latest estimates the disease has been confirmed in 18 per cent of Ugandan adults.' (BBC1 2100, 23 February 1988)

reflected in some of the audience newsgame reports. One group, for example, simply held up the photograph of black people as a visual symbol of Africa while declaring: 'This country [Britain] could be as badly affected as those abroad' (Women with children at a playground). Such reports reveal underlying assumptions: that the black photograph can represent 'Africa', that we can take it for granted that AIDS is rife 'over there', and that this is not significant in itself but only as a warning to the British public of what could happen here. They also illustrate the extent to which audiences may absorb and recall not only the content of news bulletins, but their structure and techniques, in spite of people's protests that they 'don't pay much attention to the news' or 'can't remember anything about AIDS'.

There are striking similarities between audience understandings of 'African AIDS' and contemporary television reports. The extent to which people can reconstruct media accounts, as well as the extent to which they believe those accounts, is a testament to the power of the media.

Audience Distrust of the Media

It is not simply that all these people uncritically absorb, recall and accept every aspect of media coverage in general or even AIDS coverage in particular. On the contrary, some research participants were critical of theories which were closer to home than Africa. For example, one participant reacted angrily to the suggestions that AIDS was 'a male disease', asserting that such a comment was 'Unfair. What if a woman started it?' (SACRO clients). Similarly, in a group of Scottish prisoners one man protested against the idea that AIDS was common in Edinburgh:

> That's people just starting to label. That's like us saying 'Oh no, It's all that Edinburgh mob that's got it', if you're from Glasgow, or 'all that Perth mob' or 'all that Dundee mob'. . . . They're all riddled there, but nobody in *here* is riddled with it. (Prisoners)

These white, Scottish men recognized statements about AIDS being a 'male' disease or being common in Edinburgh as carrying connotations of stigma and blame, but were not critical of similar statements which were applied to Africa.

In addition to challenging specific stories about the origins of HIV, some people declared that they were sceptical about the validity of all media reports. For some participants such scepticism arose because of personal experience of events which were later reported, and distorted, in the media. There was the mother of a sick child whose case was reported in the local press:

> Well, I've a wee boy with a heart condition and there was a report put into the paper about . . . this great operation he's had and how great he's going to be. . . . [But] some days I have to carry him to school all, [the coverage was] 'this is wonderful' and I felt like an idiot. . . . So I don't believe anything that goes in black and white . . . I thought if they can do that with him what can they do with other things? (Women with children at a playgroup, Group 2)

Some prison officers expressed similar scepticism because of their concern about media misrepresentations of their profession.

> *Resp. 1:* My granny asked if I've beaten up any prisoners yet. . . .
> *Resp. 2:* Because that's the media coverage, . . . the big bad prison officer is always beating prisoners up and then. . . .
> *Resp. 1:* My granny thinks I beat up prisoners. . . .
> (Prison staff, Group 4)

Similarly, a group of police officers stated that they were wary of what they read in the press because they knew how stories could be distorted in media accounts. One officer said that reporting of the Broadwater Farm riots had given the impression that the violence was very widespread, but he had been present in Tottenham as part of the police operation and knew that 'a couple of streets up a bit there was nothing.' One of his colleagues then gave an example of why he was sceptical about media reporting: 'I remember I was at the Old Bailey with a rape/abduction job and I was reading a report in the *Sun* and it was only in the very last bit of the report that I realised that it was a case I was involved in' (Police staff).

This group based their critique of media reporting on personal experience and generalized this critique to other subjects. Yet neither the readiness of some research participants to take issue with ideas about the prevalence or origin of AIDS when they were closer to home, nor the general scepticism of others about the media led these same people to doubt the veracity of 'African AIDS'. The police workers quoted above went on to explain their view of Africa:

Resp. 1: They all go round doing it with one another, don't they, I mean it's accepted. . . .

Resp. 2: It's a cultural way of life.

Int.: How do you know this?

Resp. 1: Again like you say we've only got the media, haven't we. None of us have got personal experience from going over there.

Resp. 2: It's pretty well catalogued from Darwin onwards.

(Police staff, Group 2)

People may profess not to 'believe anything that goes in black and white', but at the same time argue that AIDS came from, and is rife in, Africa; and say they know this because of the media. Why does this happen; why do people reject some media messages and accept others?

'Because It Fits': Audience Acceptance of 'African AIDS'

This readiness to perceive Africa as the source of HIV infection is not simply a direct response to overwhelming, or even totally consistent, media statements about AIDS, but is dependent on a broader context of reporting about Africa whereby the idea that HIV came from over there 'fits' with many white people's pre-existing images of 'the dark continent'. The notion that AIDS came from, and is widespread in, Africa or 'the Third World' falls on fertile ground by drawing upon, and feeding into, overt and covert racist agendas.

The idea that '75 million may die' 'fits' with the image of Africa as a disaster zone, whereas such decimation would be, in the words on one research partici- pant, 'unimaginable over here'. Even the media image of the person with AIDS — as thin, gaunt and wasted — 'fits' with the routine portrayal of African starvation (Watney, 1988; Patton, 1990). As one respondent put it, the enduring memory of AIDS media coverage is of 'images like Ethiopia'. The notion of AIDS as a black syndrome 'fits' with the idea of black people, and particularly black 'foreigners' and immigrants, as carriers of infection. One woman explicitly drew links between black immigration to Britain and the advent of HIV disease.

We are talking about tuberculosis and one thing and another, and we have got cures for it, maybe, but now that there's so many Asians and so forth coming over it is becoming quite rife again . . . these people are now bringing it back.' (Retired people, Group 1)[7]

Above all, media explanations of *why* AIDS came from or is common in Africa 'fit' with many white people's pre-existing understanding of 'the culture' of the continent. It is this issue which we will now explore in greater depth.

Media and Audience Explanations of AIDS in Africa: 'African Culture'

The media commonly explain HIV in Africa in terms of African culture, poverty, ignorance and promiscuity. In the period we examined, news reports on 'African AIDS' mainly gave cultural explanations for the spread of HIV infection. This allows journalists to examine the effect of poverty on health provision and to explore the 'primitive' societies in which African men won't use condoms, where 'promiscuity' is a way of life, and where people still believe in witchdoctors whose 'backward' methods help to spread HIV. The uncontrolled nature of African sexuality was a recurring theme in both news reports and audience discussions. Here ITN puts us in the picture: 'In Zambia some women's groups want to ban some of the more suggestive tribal dancing. It's one of the few admissions that a promiscuous heterosexual lifestyle is a major cause of spreading AIDS' (ITN 1745. 7 May 1987). Later the BBC tells us that the problem is the: 'traditional resistance of African men to using condoms' (BBC1 1800, 19 February 1988). Back in 1987 Channel Four News managed in two sentences to identify three ways in which primitive black Africans were 'spreading AIDS': 'The spread of AIDS is not caused by sexual promiscuity alone. . . . AIDS is encouraged by tribal doctors' traditional medicine and a widespread lack of proper medical facilities' (Channel Four News 1900, 2 February 1987).[8]

These were precisely the explanations offered by research participants. In fact, when asked to identify their source of information for believing in 'African AIDS', some participants simply gave an explanation for *why* AIDS was common in Africa rather than identifying a source. African values were seen as militating against the practice of safer sex. According to one white civil engineer: 'I'd heard that on a radio documentary . . . it's a macho thing, they [black men] won't use condoms' (Engineers). In addition, black people were seen as ignorant. As one prison officer declared: 'They're ignorant of hygiene. They've got lower intelligence at this end of the world' (Prison officers).

Above all, AIDS is associated with, and blamed on, an African sexuality which is presented as primitive and perverse, and associated with homosexuality and bestiality. One police officer argued that it made sense that AIDS came from Africa and was also a homosexual disease because homosexuality started off with 'The abominable crime of buggery . . . sorry, with animal bestiality. Now there are some very primitive people in Africa . . . and [AIDS] is alleged to have originated from practices which were a bit extreme' (Police staff, Group 1).

The idea that black people have sex with animals was also mentioned in groups of janitors, prison officers and ex-prisoners. Sometimes this theory was explicitly linked to media statements about Green Monkeys being a source of HIV.

You could say it starts off with the coloured people in Africa having it off with monkeys. (Prisoners, Group 4)

Coloured people have been know to have intercourse with anything. (Janitors)

Resp. 1: Tell us, how did it all start, I heard it was a guy had a thing with a gorilla.

Resp. 2: I heard it was a guy had sex with a bull.

Resp. 3: I heard it was a guy in Africa or something.

Resp. 1: It was just because of those black mother-fuckers from abroad, man.

Resp. 3: Had sex with a gorilla or a monkey, something like that anyway, that's why I say it was the pakis that brought it here

(SACRO clients, Group 1)

Even when not making outright allegations about black bestiality in its literal sense, other participants made it clear that they thought that AIDS was common in Africa because of the distinct (and inferior) social/sexual behaviour of black people. According to one group of white retired men and women, AIDS is common in Africa because of 'low moral standards and promiscuity . . . the Africans treat sex completely differently from the white man.'

M1: Sexual activity is not confined to one person. I mean they're promiscuous aren't they?

F1: By nature.

M2: It's their norm.

M1: They run around . . . they don't mind how many male partners they have, a women will have children by about 5 different partners, it's extraordinary. . . . It's an extraordinary set up, you need to see it to believe it.

(Retired people, Group 3)

Participants in other groups made comments such as:

They have sex all the time there. . . . They're sharing wives. (Prisoners, Group 4)

There are high amounts of prostitution in these countries. (Prison staff, Group 2)

They seem to sleep within families, i.e., fathers with children, etc. (Police staff, Group 1)

Often different notions were combined to identify Africa as an inevitable hot bed of sexuality transmitted diseases. A group of women residents on the same Glasgow estate, for example, all agreed that AIDS started in Africa because: 'They're married young' and become mature and sexually active at an early age, 'about 7' — not to mention the fact that: 'the men can have as many wives as they like' and 'there's a high risk of child prostitution in all these African countries. I seen that on "World in Action".'

It is not just that many whites are predisposed to believe that Africans *behave* in a way which spreads HIV, but that blackness and AIDS are equated in their minds. Both are associated with sexual deviance and stigmatized as dirty and alien, and simultaneously pitiful and threatening. Just as AIDS was explicitly characterized as 'The Gay Plague', implicitly it is also 'The Black Death'. According to some young people in intermediate treatment, for example, AIDS *must* have originated in Africa.

Resp. 1: Look at all the famine over there, all the disease coming off the dead cows and all that they die and all that.

Resp. 2: That's just like dirtiness and things like that.

Resp. 3: Dirtiness.

Resp. 2: Filthy.

Resp. 1: Blackness.

Int.: Blackness? What about it?

Resp. 3: It's black.

Resp. 1: Black, blackness, it's black, that's what I mean it's dirty.

Resp. 2: It's just disgusting.

(Young people in intermediate treatment)

Many people are predisposed to accept the AIDS-Africa link because white Western culture, often through the media, constructs images of Africa and of black people as poverty stricken and disease ridden, as immigrants threatening the purity and stability of white society, and as primitives with a dangerous, destructive and uncontrolled sexuality.[9] Some of these themes are implicit (and some explicit) in media coverage of 'African AIDS', but people also drew on a wide range of other media and non-media sources. In talking about why they associated AIDS with Africa, people referred to sources such as a 'World in Action' documentary about Africa, famine relief advertisements, a poster showing evolution from monkey to man and a whole range of accounts of Africa 'pretty well catalogued from Darwin onwards'.

Media Can Cut Across Prior Political Beliefs

It was not only people who articulated explicitly racist views on Africa who had come to accept key information or assumptions about the links between AIDS and Africa or black people. In some cases research participants had accepted this information *in spite* of their own expressed political views and they became uncomfortable with this once challenged by other members of the group. One group of market researchers, for example, wrote a newsgame report which identifies gays, prostitutes, injecting drug users and 'the Afro/Caribbean community' as high risk groups. It was only after re-reading the text that they expressed reservations about some of their assumptions:

Resp. 1: [Our news bulletin] suggested that the Afro/Caribbean community in this country was responsible for spread which isnae really true. . . . There is a problem in Africa of course but whether that makes the Afro/Caribbean community in this country any more at risk than the general population, I don't know, I don't think it does.

Resp. 2: As far as I'm aware, no.

Resp. 3: No, it doesnae.

Resp. 1: So we probable made a boob there.

The debate about whether or not AIDS was common in Africa, and if so *why* this was the case, was explored in depth during a discussion among three NACRO workers, two of whom were black (Resp. 2 and 3) and one of whom was white (Resp. 1). The offices where these men worked were hung with positive images of black historical, cultural and political figures such as Bob Marley, Martin Luther King and Nelson Mandela. The white worker asserted that AIDS was widespread in Africa and commented:

> *Resp. 1:* I seem to remember seeing various documentaries about it saying it's wiping out whole sort of villages, . . . some of the villages, it's a cultural thing that the men sleep around.

The two black workers, however, vehemently disagreed with this explanation. One on them declared:

> *Resp. 2:* I think it's a misconception that there are people that are like uncontrolled . . . I believe the media uses that conception they bung it in people's heads for years and years and when they want to they just feed back into it.

The white man then attempted to resolve the tension between his politics, the views of his colleagues and the information supplied by the media by qualifying his answer:

> *Resp. 1:* People say AIDS is prevalent in Africa but it might be only in *certain* countries or even in certain parts. To say that AIDS as a whole is present in Africa as a whole, I'm sure that's not true. And this thing I was saying about, this certain tribe, this was just a certain programme that I saw . . . I meant to clarify that it was just in that *particular* community, not for the *whole* of Africa, you know.

His colleagues went on to say:

> *Resp. 2:* Well it's not just TV. As I said, through the educational system, the history books where the lie has been going on so long, when the media wants to, they can tap back into that lie, because it's come out of books. You know books, you think 'fact' OK, so naturally if the media is saying this and you remember from your school days what the books said, then it's true.
>
> *Resp. 3:* It's the whole thing about the Third World, you know, the image of the Third World is somehow, they've got a bad name, they're not civilized or they need to catch up with Western ideas.

The tensions were finally resolved by the white man's acceptance of this alternative perspective elaborated by his colleagues:

> *Resp. 1:* I would agree. I was saying about history . . . all I remember from my history about Africa is it's where slaves come from

> and people live in mud huts in tribes, you know. That's the
> sort of image you get of what African life is about.

Such images of Africa are deeply embedded in white Western culture, being
endemic in history books, science, literature, films, documentaries, famine relief
adverts and in the news. But the power of the media is neither absolute nor all-
pervasive; the 'fit' is not completely watertight, and the acceptance of the African-
AIDS association is not inevitable. A few people rejected the story of 'African
AIDS', and it is to the reasons for those rejections that we now turn.

Audience Rejection of 'African AIDS'

This section explores seven main factors which influenced people to reject the
Africa-AIDS association:

> personal contact with alternative information from trusted individuals or or-
> ganizations;
>
> white people making links with their own experience of being scapegoated in
> the AIDS story (e.g. white lesbians or gay men);
>
> direct personal experience of conditions in Africa;
>
> exposure to alternative media accounts;
>
> receptiveness to alternative origin theories which 'fit' with another way of
> understanding the world;
>
> awareness of racism;
>
> structural position, in particular, being black.

Personal Contact.   We have already shown how some research participants modified their opinions during the course of discussion — after reflecting on their own
assumptions or being challenged by colleagues. Other people reported incidents
prior to participating in the discussion group which has caused them to alter their
opinion. One gay man said he used to think HIV came from Africa but had
changed his mind at a Terrence Higgins Trust (THT) conference where a black
woman criticized the Trust for their leaflets saying AIDS came from Africa, and
the THT 'admitted that they threw that in without actually knowing. They're not
awfully sure where it came from.'

Making Links with One's Own Oppression (as a White Person).   It was not simply
exposure to such alternative information which made this gay man change his
mind but the fact that people he trusted (the THT workers) accepted the woman's
point and apologized for their error in promoting the African origin idea. In
addition, he could readily comprehend how the African origin theory could feed
into racism and linked his understanding of this directly to his own experience of
oppression as a gay man.

> [It's] the same with that AIDS being spread into the heterosexual popu-
> lation as though it's sort of 'sewer of homosexuals' are starting this dis-
> ease and now are infecting the general population and its *our* fault or *blacks*
> or whoever you can blame, prostitutes' fault. (Gay men, Group 2)

Direct Personal Experience. Another form of more direct personal experience was related by a Tanzanian research participant: he did not accept the Western media's cataclysmic scenarios about AIDS in Africa because he knew the places they were talking about: 'The Western press focuses on AIDS in Africa, as if you'd just visited Dar es Salaam or Nairobi you'd find bodies, people dying in the streets — which is not the case' (African journalists' group).[10]

Exposure to Alternative Media Information. Other participants rejected the African origin theory as a result of watching one particular documentary — 'Monkey Business' — which attacked the African origin theory and suggested that the virus could have originated in a laboratory.[11] This programme was screened during the period of our fieldwork and was cited in some of the subsequent groups to challenge the idea that the virus came from Africa. Several participants in the group of teachers, for example, had watched 'Monkey Business', and some of the ideas presented in this programme had confirmed earlier accounts which they recalled as 'rumours', although they were not accepted uncritically.

When one teacher asserted as fact that AIDS came from Africa, her colleagues commented that this was 'just theory'.

Resp. 1:   There's some evidence now that it's not from Africa at all and it's perhaps a racist thing to start involving Africans in it.

Int.:   What evidence is that?

Resp. 1:   I saw it on Channel 4 a couple of weeks ago.

Int.:   What did you think of that programme?

Resp. 1:   It was very one-sided but I mean if it was true then, the evidence was there but. . . .

Resp. 2:   The first thing I heard was the theory that it was designed in the laboratory and it was tested on monkeys — and this was a long time ago and it was all sort of suppositions — and the monkeys had escaped. This is it, it's all supposition but if that was all sort of a wishy-washy rumour that was going around 5 or 6 years ago then why is it now that people are still concentrating on this and taking it seriously?

(Teachers)

One retired man, who had also watched 'Monkey Business' a few days before the research session, referred to it in detail. His acceptance of the position taken by 'Monkey Business' was influenced both by his consideration of the evidence presented on the programme and by his view of the power of the media to manipulate public opinion.

Resp. 1:   I don't accept that glib response from United States that it couldn't have originated here, it must have originated in these primitive tribes — the Green Monkey Theory.

Int.:   Why don't you accept that?

Resp. 1:   Because newspapers can manipulate public opinion. . . . They went to the source, where some people were claiming it originated among these so-called primitive tribes, where there's no evidence of AIDS at all.

(Retired people, Group 1)

Receptiveness to Another Origin Theory Which 'Fits'. The African origin theory is, of course, not the only theory which 'fits' with many Westerners' understandings of the world. The idea that HIV was created in a laboratory 'fits' with popular perceptions of 'mad scientists' who lose control of their inventions or have deliberately evil and unnatural intentions: 'They're experimenting with all sorts and doing all sorts, they're transferring brains and things' (Women with children at playgroup, Group 1).[12]

One of the teachers who had watched 'Monkey Business' commented that, in spite of reservations about the programme, the theory that the virus originated in a laboratory was credible because: 'the US government has nevertheless spent millions of pounds grafting retroviruses with leukaemia viruses and there's bound to be something strange happening from these things'.

In another group, when one gay man referred to a story about 'Americans releasing the virus', another said he believed this was 'entirely possible': 'I think the Americans are probably capable of doing such things' (Gay men). Similarly, a drug user in a drug rehabilitation centre commented: 'My personal opinion is it was germ warfare. They are still producing them, the Russians and no doubt the Americans as well, and don't know about the British. How do we know they've not released something like that and just lost control?'

The view of HIV as a laboratory invention 'fits' with what people know about other 'man-made' disasters; anthrax and myxomatosis were mentioned by research participants. The laboratory theory also 'fits' with some people's understanding of government secrecy and corruption and officials' disregard both for the truth and for public health; Bhopal and Chernobyl were given as illustrations here. A group of Glasgow women, for example, discussed the accident at the Chernobyl nuclear power station and its effects on Scottish farmers and consumers.

> *Resp. 1:* They've got some farms that still can't sell their things, they're still killing their cattle, their sheep, you name it. The grass — the radiation affects the grass, the earth, we're eating potatoes and carrots and whatnot.
>
> *Resp. 2:* They said it was alright and then later they said it could have been in the rain, it could have been carried.
>
> *Resp. 1:* They tell you a lot of rubbish.
>
> *Resp. 2:* Even Salmonella in the eggs that's another theory — how they covered that up.
>
> *Resp. 1:* Also, how many of you would let your children go in the water on a beach near a nuclear power station? I mean I wouldn't.

This reflected and reinforced a general distrust of public information.

> *Resp. 1:* [The government] tell too many lies and you can't trust them for nothing.
>
> *Resp. 2:* They tell you what they want to tell you.
>
> (Women with children at a playgroup, Group 1)

Awareness of Racism. Many white participants were aware that theories about 'African AIDS' could be interpreted as, or contribute to, racism. Several groups rejected using the photograph of black people in their news report at all because they could see only negative connotations in it.

> We rejected this one [the photograph] of the black people because we actually thought it was a bit racist as well to assume that the origins of AIDS was with black people and we thought if we put that one across then people would be racist against blacks saying they've all got AIDS. (Students, Group 2)

This awareness of racism meant that in some groups participants who asserted the African origins theory were quickly challenged by friends or colleagues:

> *Resp. 1*: I think somebody brought it over from Africa, you get it there.
> *Resp. 2*: Shut up you.
> *Resp. 1*: What?
> *Resp. 2*: Blame the Africans.
> *Resp. 3*: Racism straight away!
> (Young people in intermediate treatment)[13]

Structural Position.   The single factor common to research participants who most clearly rejected the association of AIDS with Africa was that they were black. The importance of this factor was most clearly demonstrated in our work with two groups of ex-prisoners in resettlement schemes — one in Glasgow, the other in London. Both groups were largely male and working-class. However, the Glasgow group was all white and the London one mostly black. While comments such as '[It was] they black bastards that brought AIDS over here,' were common in the Glasgow group, some of the London group produced a tongue-in-cheek news bulletin which gave quite a different message:

> This is Trevor McDoughnut with the News at Ten. . . . Mr Norman Fowler [who] we spoke to earlier on today has told us that one of the ideas that AIDS may have come from is the Pentagon, a secret plan instigated by. . . . [Making sound of interference on the TV screen and then putting on a heavy American accent] . . . .My name is General Lee Eisenhower and I would like to say that the Pentagon has nothing at all to do with the AIDS problem. It has nothing to do at all with us, I deny it strongly, I mean I've never been to Africa myself so there's no way that AIDS could have been instigated by us. I mean, who knows, I mean it's not my fault that they're catching it through some food that we put — oops sorry. [Returning to voice of a newscaster] Here we have Dr Tefal. AIDS — it has been brought to our attention by a certain Sergeant Pepper, has been instigated into Africa into America and into different other countries by the Pentagon as a means to control world population. In the year 2500 it has been estimated that there will be a population explosion — too many people will be living so they've decided to cut down on it. (NACRO clients)

This 'news bulletin' caused much laughter and offered an implicit critique of the 'African AIDS' story. It seems clear that the production of this critique is related to structural rather than individual factors. As the person who read this bulletin said when asked why he did not believe that AIDS came from Africa: 'I am biased on the subject, right because I'm a black man.'[14]

However, structural position, awareness of racism, understanding other kinds of oppression or exposure to other arguments do not necessarily lead to criticism of images of Africa or 'African AIDS'. Some research participants reported that other black friends and relations accepted the African AIDS story and, within the groups, there were examples where people's own experience of oppression, their awareness of racism or their personal experience clearly did not lead them to reject the idea that AIDS either came from, or was rife in, Africa. A young white lesbian, for example, reiterated the idea that AIDS spread from Africa in order to absolve gay men from blame. Her news report argued:

AIDS is said to have spread through the homosexuals in America and a lot of the practices they participate in whereas in fact it could have originated from Green Monkeys in Africa, spreading from the heterosexual population over to America. (Lesbians, Group 2)

Very few respondents cited personal experience of being in Africa as a source of information about AIDS. However, the retired, white, heterosexual couple who had waxed lyrical about African promiscuity and concluded, 'you have to see it to believe it', had in fact visited South Africa. They used this experience to reinforce their prejudices and their belief in media versions of AIDS in Africa. This couple were part of a group of retired people in Kent and both were *Daily Telegraph* readers. They were confident in their knowledge that AIDS was common in Africa because:

We heard it actually from someone who was connected with the blood bank in Durban who was telling us about the tests they did on this school and out of a hundred, about a hundred tests, four were positive and one was the teacher. When you've got that sort of problem you really are in it up to here.

Awareness that the African origin theory could be interpreted as racist is not the same as accepting that it is. In a group of white staff in a London police station (the group in which one police officer had referred to the 'primitive' and 'extreme' sexual practices of Africa) a member of the administrative staff in the station explained why her newsgame team had not used the picture of black people: 'That's where is started — in the black provinces, but we didn't go in to it. You've got to watch that in case people think it's racist' (Police staff, Group 1). This concern that propounding the 'fact' that HIV started in the 'black provinces' might be *seen* as racist, rather than recognizing that the way it would be used would actually have been racist is instructive. This worry is partially explained by the case of one black police recruit who resigned from this particular station, alleging that he had been subjected to systematic racial abuse. A number of participants in this group made (half-joking) statements that they would have to be careful what they said.

Conclusions

Our research shows both the power of the media and the pervasiveness of stock white cultural images of black Africa; it is easy to believe that Africa is a reservoir of HIV infection because 'it fits'. Journalists draw on these cultural assumptions when they produce reports on AIDS and Africa. But in so doing they are helping to reproduce and legitimize them. News reports often treat black Africa as an undifferentiated whole, use images of blackness to represent the disease, and display a cavalier attitude to statistics about the scale of the disaster. In addition, news reporters' explanations of African AIDS routinely conceptualize the problem in terms of an 'African culture'. The problem is 'traditional sexual values' or 'traditional tribal medicine', as if white Western culture had nothing to do with HIV transmission in Britain, as if white Western (heterosexual) men never resisted using condoms, and as if white Western medicine never infected thousands of people through contaminated blood products. It is almost as if AIDS in Africa is something to do with Africanness and blackness itself.

Having said this, it is clear that the media are neither an all-powerful conduit for dominant ideas nor is their output completely one-dimensional. Alternative media information does exist, and is important in facilitating access to different ways of understanding the world. We also saw how personal experience, people's own structural position, experience of oppression, or understanding of racism were all factors which meant that people could be critical of the media, although they did not guarantee that they were.

People's understandings are not entirely defined and confined by the media, and their ideas may change according to how they interpret new information. In our research sessions we witnessed people reassessing their ideas in view of inconsistencies thrown up during the discussion or after being told of other evidence by another participant, as well as in response to the pressure of what was assumed to be 'known' by the rest of the group.

Perhaps what is most important is that these openings exist, and that the winning of consent for dominant views is not simply given but is an ongoing process. Carrying out research such as that described here allows us to examine the links between media content and audience beliefs; it also enables a strategic assessment of the gaps and weaknesses of powerful ideas, images and systems of thought.

Notes

1 This study is part of the AIDS Media Research Project funded by the ESRC (Award Number A44250006). We would like to acknowledge the help of our colleagues — Peter Beharrell, Lorna Brown and Kevin Williams — and the grant-holders — Mick Bloor, John Eldridge, Sally MacIntyre and Greg Philo. In addition, thanks to Frank Mosson, Lesley Parker and Linda Steele for assistance with early coding and content analysis.
2 The main bulletins examined were the early and late evening news programmes on ITN (1740/1745 and 2200), BBC1 (1800 and 2100) and the Channel Four news.
3 Both authors of this paper are white. It is clear that this common factor played some role in our research sessions, as did our different class backgrounds, gender,

sexual identities and national origins. We hope to discuss these issues in a later paper.

4   We did find examples of people who believed that HIV was widespread in Africa but did not associate this 'fact' with the origins of AIDS, and others who were unsure where HIV came from but saw that question as irrelevant. They clearly distinguished between the two issues, suspending belief about where the virus came from, but perceiving the issue of the world-wide distribution of the virus as a crucial basis for action.

5   The idea that HIV is a problem that affects 'other people', 'over there' — literally and figuratively — puts distance between the audience and the potential victims of infection. One gay man had first heard about AIDS as a problem in San Francisco and Africa. He commented: 'it's just like you are aware of malnutrition in East Africa, you are aware of the floods in Bangladesh, but if it's not relevant to you, you store it back in your mind, but it's just there for reference purposes' (Gay men, Group 1). This has direct practical consequences. One HIV antibody positive prisoner described his bitterness about the fact that he had not been aware that AIDS was a problem in Britain around the time he became infected: 'I'd heard of it, but not over here, I'd heard of it like from America and Africa and things like that. Like at the time when I caught it and most of my mates caught it nothing had been said about it being over here' (Prisoners, Group 1).

6   Treichler argues that photographs of AIDS in Africa:

> Reinforce what we think we already know about AIDS in those regions: frail, wasting bodies in gloomy clinics; small children in rackety cribs; the prostitute in red. Photographs in a 1986 *Newsweek* story on AIDS in Africa depict the 'Third Worldness' of its health care system: in Tanzania, a man with AIDS lies hospitalised on a plain cot with none of the high tech paraphernalia of US representation; a widely reprinted photograph shows six emaciated patients in a Uganda AIDS ward, two in cots, four on mats on the floor; rarely are physicians shown. A story on AIDS in Brazil carries similar non-technological images. In contrast, African publications often run photos of African scientists and physicians, and among the photographs in a 1987 story on AIDS in the Brazilian equivalent of *Newsweek* is one of a fully equipped operating theatre complete with masked and gowned physicians and nurses. (Treichler, 1989, p. 45)

7   Black people were explicitly blamed for AIDS by several of the groups involved in this study. Identifying Africa as a source of contagion also 'fits' with fear of, and the desire to control, black immigration. In the words of one white retired man, the African AIDS association is: 'A marvellous platform for Enoch Powell actually. He was right, dead right, we should have kept them out' (Retired people, Group 3). It also 'fits' into overtly racist attitudes and policies towards black immigrants. In their newsgame report, one team in this group of retired people conclude: 'All immigrants coming into the country from epidemic areas are to be screened for the disease before admission into the country.' This statement was greeted by another member of the group with assent: 'Yes, that's a point' (Retired people, Group 3).

8   While this was the dominant picture of AIDS in Africa, there was some news information in this period which could have been used to give a different understanding. This view sees the role of the West through the lens of its colonial history and argues that Western blaming of Africa for AIDS has more to do with racism than with medical knowledge or science. What is extraordinary about these

references is that some of them are used by the journalist as further evidence of the backwardness of black Africans; for example: 'Here, where tribal doctors still have not heard of AIDS, there are deeply rooted fears and suspicions that the West somehow wants to blame Africa for the start of the AIDS epidemic' (ITN, 2200, 7 May 1987). Noting the same phenomena among the media reports she examined, Treichler concludes:

> The notion that AIDS is an American invention is a recurrent element of the international AIDS story, yet not one easily incorporated within a Western positivist frame, in part, perhaps, because it is political, with discursive roots in the resistance to colonialism; the Western response, accordingly, attributes it to ignorance, state propaganda or psychological denial. (Treichler, 1989, p. 43)

9 Research on public perceptions of Africa conducted in the mid-1980s with young people age 14–18 reported overwhelmingly negative and condescending attitudes towards Africa. Africa was associated with poverty, hunger, dirt, suffering and crying. 'It is dirty . . . lots of flies . . . they smell.' Africa was seen as primitive and dependent on Western aid. There was a lack of understanding of the history and economic, social, political and cultural life in Africa (Van der Gaag and Nash, 1987). For further discussion of, and research on, white images of Africa, see Husband, 1975; Laishley, 1975; Philo and Lamb, 1986; Van der Gaag and Nash, 1987; Simpson, 1985.

10 It is not being argued that personal experience is necessarily the source of authentic truth, or that it will necessarily contradict the media. However, 'personal experience' is a powerful influence and rhetorical technique. Phrases such as 'I was there', 'I saw it with my own eyes', 'You have to see it to believe it' were often used in our research sessions to win consent for particular views.

11 'Monkey Business: AIDS — The Africa Story' was broadcast on Channel Four on 22 January 1990 at 11.05 p.m. The audience for programmes like this is considerably smaller than that for a television news bulletin. 'Monkey Business' was watched by 581,000 people. On the same night the audiences for the BBC's 'Nine O'clock News' and ITN's 'News at Ten' were 6,224,000 and 7,093,000 respectively (figures from BARB, 22 January 1990).

12 Patton argues that, 'When the West found itself beset by a deadly little virus of unknown origin, it sought the source elsewhere; nothing of this sort, it was argued, could have arisen in the germ-free west. So the best research minds of the western world set off on a fantastic voyage in search of the source of AIDS' (Patton, 1990, p. 29). However, the idea that HIV did originate in 'the germ-free West' does at least fit with the Western lay imagination's distrust of the scientific hocus pocus conducted in sterile laboratories.

13 Reservations about 'harping on' about the possibility that AIDS came from Africa could be independent of belief in whether or not it did in fact do so.

14 Belief in information depends partly on the perceived credibility of the source. For example, some research participants talked dismissively of information received from, or views expressed by, 'old women' (School students), 'my holier-than-thou-mother-in-law' (Playgroup) and 'comedy papers' such as *The News of the World*, *The Sun* and *The Sunday Sport*. However, the credibility ascribed to a source depends partly on whether or not it offers an expected or wanted viewpoint. For example, one white retired woman who had earlier expressed antagonism toward 'immigrants' and 'homosexuals' suddenly backed up her own argument that 'AIDS came from Africa' by declaring that this had been started by a black, gay man in a book she had read.

References

ADAMS, J. (1989) *AIDS: The HIV Myth*, London, Macmillan.
AGGLETON, P. and HOMANS, H. (Eds) (1988) *Social Aspects of AIDS*, Lewes, Falmer Press.
BOFFIN, T. and GUPTA, S. (Eds) (1988) *Ecstatic Antibodies: Resisting the AIDS Mythology*, London, Rivers Oram Press.
CHIRIMUUTA, R. and CHIRIMUUTA, R. (1989) *AIDS, Africa and Racism*, London, Free Association Books.
Critical Health (1988), 'AIDS in South Africa: Progressive Perspectives', Number 22, April, Johannesburg.
DADA, M. (1990) 'Race and the AIDS Agenda', in T. BOFFIN and S. GUPTA (Eds), *Ecstatic Antibodies: Resisting the AIDS Mythology*, London, Rivers Oram Press.
HUSBAND, C. (Ed.) (1975) *White Media and Black Britain*, London, Arrow Books.
KITZINGER, J. (1990) 'Audience Understandings of AIDS Media Messages: A Discussion of Methods', *Sociology of Health and Illness*, 12, 3, pp. 319–35.
KITZINGER, J. and MILLER, D. (1991) 'In Black and White: A Preliminary Report on the Role of the Media in Audience Understandings of "African AIDS"', MRC Working Paper No. 27, Glasgow, University of Glasgow, Medical Sociology Unit.
LAISHLEY, J. (1975) 'The Images of Blacks and Whites in the Children's Media', in C. HUSBAND (Ed.), *White Media and Black Britain*, London, Arrow Books.
MACBRIDE, S., *et al*. (1981) *Many Voices, One World: Communication and Society, Today and Tomorrow*, Report of the International Commission for the Study of Communication Problems, UNESCO, Paris, Kogan Page.
MCQUEEN, D., GORST, T., NISBET, L., ROBERTSON, B., SMITH, R. and UITENBROEK, D. (1989) *Interim Report No 1*, May/October 8, 1989 Edinburgh, RUHBC.
PATTON, C. (1990) 'Inventing "African AIDS"', *New Formations*, 10, pp. 25–39.
PHILO, G. (1990) *Seeing and Believing: The Influence of Television*, London, Routledge.
PHILO, G. and LAMB, R. (1986) *Television and the Ethiopian Famine: From Buerk to Band AID*, Prepared for UNESCO and the Canadian Film Institute, London, Television Trust for the Environment.
SABATIER, R. (1988) *Blaming Others: Prejudice, Race and World-wide AIDS*, London, Panos.
SIMPSON, A. (1985) 'Charity Begins at Home', *Ten: Eight*, 19, pp. 21–6.
SONTAG, S. (1989) *AIDS and Its Metaphors*, Harmondsworth, Penguin Books.
TREICHLER, P. (1989) 'AIDS and HIV Infection in the Third World: A First World Chronicle', in B. KRUGER, and P. MARIANI (Eds), *Discussions in Contemporary Culture: Remaking History*, 4, pp. 31–86.
VAN DER GAAG, N. and NASH, C. (1987) *Images of Africa: The UK Report*, Oxford, Oxfam.
WARWICK, I., AGGLETON, P. and HOMANS, H. (1988) 'Young People's Health Beliefs and AIDS', in P. AGGLETON and H. HOMANS (Eds), *Social Aspects of AIDS*, Lewes, Falmer Press.
WATNEY, S. (1988) 'Missionary Positions: AIDS, "Africa" and Race', *Differences: A Feminist Journal of Cultural Studies*, 1, 1, pp. 83–100.

4   The Politics of AIDS in Britain and Germany

Richard Freeman

The comparative analysis of AIDS policy-making is still in its infancy. Country case studies are few,[1] and comparisons between them even fewer.[2] Comparative study offers an opportunity to learn not only about responses to AIDS, but also something about the policy contexts in which strategies of prevention in health are formulated. More widely still, as Weeks (1989, p. 13) has observed, 'AIDS has . . . provided important insights into the complexities of policy formation in pluralist societies.'

Elsewhere, Moerkerk and Aggleton (1990) have bravely, and uniquely, attempted a typology of AIDS prevention strategies in Europe. Their modelling — of pragmatic, political, biomedical and emergent responses — is not my concern here. I am interested in their placing together of (then West) Germany, the UK and Sweden in the same 'political' category. This refers to AIDS policy as having been developed in accordance with what is politically possible or politically desirable in a given country, and to AIDS strategies having been defined or even dictated by governments. Categorization of this kind is not wholly satisfactory since it obscures important differences of emphasis, of process and of detail. It is, moreover, descriptive rather than explanatory. Nevertheless, it begs useful further questions: what are the politics of AIDS policy-making?

This chapter examines the politics of AIDS policy-making in Britain and Germany.[3] It distinguishes two levels of difference beneath a superficial similarity in the patterns of their respective policy responses: first, a difference in the process of the production of policy within government; and, second, a difference in the relationship between government and AIDS service organizations in the voluntary sector (ASOs).[4] It begins, by way of introduction, with a historical overview of the period 1982–90.

The discussion is based on research material gathered during 1990 in Cologne, Bonn, Berlin, Manchester and London, including government and parliamentary documents, the policy statements of AIDS-related institutions and agencies, and secondary social scientific literature. Additional material is taken from a number of research interviews held with individuals whose experience made them especially qualified to discuss policy-making in respect of HIV and AIDS. They included civil servants, health officials, managers of AIDS agencies and social scientists. They were selected to represent both government and administration and the statutory and voluntary service sectors, and to include the range of local, regional and national levels of organization. Some of this interview data has been used here in anonymized form.

Before the material proper is considered, it is important to establish the comparability of these case studies in respect of HIV/AIDS epidemiology. Both Germany and the UK are recognized 'Type 1' countries: the HIV/AIDS epidemic emerged among gay and bisexual men in the period after 1981, being seen by the mid-1980s in drug injecting populations. The German AIDS case rate per million population has been slightly higher: 8.8 compared with 6.9 for the UK at the end of June 1986; 23.0 in Germany and 18.9 in the UK at the end of September 1987, according to WHO figures. Case numbers in Germany, though weighted toward Berlin, were and are more evenly distributed among the major cities of the Federal Republic than in the UK; in Britain case prevalence is strongly centred on the capitals London and Edinburgh. The prevalence of HIV infection in each country can only be estimated, but the argument here proceeds from the assumption that levels of infection, or even fairly precise estimates of prevalence, mattered less to policy-makers and politicians in 1986–87 than a theoretically plausible sense of a generalized threat to their heterosexual populations.

The primary contrast between the two countries is structural and organizational, between respective political, social policy and health care systems, and it is this which is of particular interest here. Germany is a federal state; welfare, though regulated by the state at federal, regional and local levels, is provided by essentially private organizations (the *Verbände*).[5] The UK has a much more strongly centralized state, which plays a key role in the funding and delivery of welfare; this is epitomized by its National Health Service, which is subdivided hierarchically into Regional and District Health Authorities. How, then, do such markedly different systems respond to a similar epidemiological threat?

AIDS: A Comparative History

For the sake of ordering the analysis offered here, three phases of response to HIV/AIDS can be distinguished: the nascent response (roughly 1982–85), crisis (1986–87) and administration (1988–90). In keeping with the subsequent discussion, the detail is slightly biased toward the ASOs and intersectoral relations.

The Nascent Response 1982–85

First diagnoses of AIDS were reported in the UK and in West Germany in 1982. In the absence of any other form of protective response, and in fear of the reverse, the first AIDS self-help groups (the AIDS-Hilfen) were set up by gay men in Munich and Berlin in 1983, and in Cologne, Hamburg and Frankfurt during 1984; in London the Terrence Higgins Trust was also formed in 1983. At the same time, work on AIDS was included in programmes of clinical research sponsored by the UK's Medical Research Council and the German Federal Ministry of Research and Technology.

Perhaps reflecting the newness of AIDS as a disease category, and the corresponding uncertainties which it aroused, policy communities in both countries were unusually open during 1984–85. A meeting took place in Düsseldorf in March 1985, for example, between federal and regional health officials, clinicians, sexologists and representatives of the German National Institute of Health, the Federal Centre for Health Education and of the *AIDS-Hilfen*. The *Deutsche AIDS-Hilfe* was formally constituted as an umbrella organization of local AIDS-Hilfe groups in December 1985. More or less simultaneously, AIDS policy lobbies in London fostered among genito-urinary consultants and gay men (organizationally focused on the Terrence Higgins Trust) began to coalesce around the public health interest at the governmental Department of Health (see Berridge and Strong, 1990). An Expert Advisory Group on AIDS met for the first time in January 1985, and the Department of Health set up its own internal AIDS Unit at the end of the year.

In many respects local and regional developments preceded central government action. The Berlin senate formed its *AIDS-Task-Force* in 1985, Hamburg set up a coordinating office for AIDS policy in early 1986, while public health offices in Munich, Bremen and Cologne became established as focal points of local policy organization. In the UK there was early activity in Oxford, Brighton, Sheffield and elsewhere during 1985–86. Manchester City Council established an AIDS Working Party in January 1986, which published a policy statement in November that same year.

Crisis 1986–87

During 1986 and 1987 AIDS was elevated from an administrative, departmental or even merely local concern to an issue of national politics. It is at this point that the patterns of policy-making diverge. While policy communities were still relatively open, the British response remained low-key and informal while that in Germany became public and confrontational. In Britain, in 1986, government circulars were issued to health authorities and local government bodies in May and July respectively, asking them to set up local action groups on AIDS and giving advice to staff working with those who may have been infected with HIV or who had AIDS. A cabinet committee on AIDS was convened in October, funds were committed to a mass media campaign of public education on HIV and AIDS in November, a National AIDS Helpline was opened in December and an information leaflet on AIDS was distributed by the Department of Health to all households in January 1987.

A similar flurry of policy activity in Germany was delayed by the federal elections imminent in January 1987. Here the issue was escalated by fundamental political conflict over the role of law in prevention. A liberal line of widespread education complemented and supported by voluntary testing, and favoured by the social-catholic wing of the major party of government, the conservative Christian Democrats (CDU), was opposed by an authoritarian position, based on the criminalization of HIV transmission and the forcible testing of 'those suspected of being infectious', which had originated in the Bavarian Ministry of the Interior. This conflict was used by the Bavarian Christian Socialists (CSU) as a lever of influence in the coalition negotiations of the incoming government which took place in March between the Christian Democrats, themselves and the liberal Free Democrats (FDP). The outcome of these events was that the government committed itself to a liberal policy stance, based on public education, voluntary testing and counselling, setting up coordinating units at the Ministry of Health and the Federal Health Office (cf. BMJFFG, 1990).[6] The regional states (the *Länder*) fell into line behind Bonn by the end of the month at a special joint meeting of health ministers,[7] leaving Bavaria isolated. Bavaria published its own legal-repressive measures in May.[8] In June the *Deutsche AIDS-Hilfe* published an important position statement, the *Memorandum* (Deutsche AIDS-Hilfe (1987), which laid out a dual policy of self-help by, and solidarity with, those affected by HIV and AIDS.[9] In October, as something of a political compromise, a compulsory system of anonymous notification by testing laboratories of positive tests for HIV was introduced.

At the same time, health education in both countries was becoming more politically protected, if not directly managed. Increased AIDS funding for health education bodies (the sums involved were similar in the two countries) was linked to increased control by their respective departments of health. The institution of the AIDS Coordination Unit at the German Ministry of Health in October 1987, for example, is felt to have limited the previous autonomy in respect of AIDS enjoyed by the Federal Centre for Health Education. The UK's Health Education Authority, which was accorded responsibility for the government's AIDS campaign also in October 1987, had been reconstituted in April of that year from the Health Education Council, and was brought more closely under the direction of the Department of Health. Governments' commitment to health education was supported by a network of consensus-building advisory bodies — a National AIDS Advisory Council and a parliamentary Commission of Inquiry on AIDS. In Germany the *Nationaler AIDS-Beirat* performed functions similar in effect to those of the UK's Expert Advisory Group on AIDS, the Social Services Select Committee and the All-Party Parliamentary Group on AIDS.

Policy Administration 1988–90

In Germany the AIDS *Modellprogramme* were established under the auspices of the coalition agreement, and given short-term federal funding for the period 1987–91 (see BMJFFG, 1990). Major provisions included the financing, from federal resources, of a specialist AIDS post (professionally a physician, psychologist or social worker) at all 309 local public health offices. A further forty-seven street worker posts were also established across the country, as were specialized counselling and research programmes. These were supported by regional state programmes. Berlin set up its *Schoolworkerprogramm* in 1987 (see Hachmann, Langemann and Bargstedt, 1990), and a *Youth-Work-Program* was established in NRW in March 1988 (Franzkowiak, 1989).

The National AIDS Trust, a fundraising and coordinating body for the UK voluntary sector, was set up in May 1987. Guidance from the Department of Health in 1986 had suggested that District Health Authorities establish Standing Action Groups on AIDS; in February 1989 the Department of Health asked that HIV Prevention Coordinations be appointed in each District. By 1990, in both countries, the thrust of AIDS policy had reverted to the local management of locally constructed programmes.[10]

Governing the AIDS Crisis

The German debate over responses to AIDS was dominated by law rather than medicine, the issue being the applicability of the Federal Epidemic Law (the *Bundeseuchengesetz*) to AIDS. Public health and clinical medicine alike appeared divided; the *AIDS-Hilfen*, to whom both federal and regional funds were already committed, lobbied at both levels for solidarity with those affected by AIDS and for community-oriented approaches to prevention. In Germany political uncertainty produced a conflict between authoritarian and liberal ideologies; in the UK, to witness a paradox, uncertainty seems to have increased political reliance on professional knowledge and expertise (Day and Klein, 1989; but c.f. Berridge and Strong, 1990). Ministers willingly deferred to professional medical advice, which ran against compulsory screening and in favour of prevention through health education.

Government interest can be perceived to have been similar in both cases; the first inclination of each was to evade demands for radical intervention, whether legal or social, and to devolve responsibility for the management of crisis into the realms of the individual and local, beyond its own sphere of action. It is in this sense that responses to AIDS may be deemed to have been 'political' rather than pragmatic, having as much to do with the negotiation of power and responsibility as with the practicalities of 'solving the problem'.

In a complementary way the British policy response reflected the administrative organization of medicine in Britain, in which the Department of Health acts in effect as the Department of the National Health Service. Following the relocation of the public health function from the local authority to the District Health Authority, which culminated in implementation of the recommendations of the Acheson Report of 1988, responses to AIDS were shaped by medicine's tendency to think in terms of the individual and the limited capacity of the NHS to develop strategies for health promotion which go beyond health education.

German AIDS policy reflected a federal, much less centralized or statist politics which allows greater access to minority groups. Both the formal access of CSU and the informal access of the *AIDS-Hilfen* to the political process were made possible and were sustained by German federalism. The federal government, without policy responsibility for public health (which is devolved to the regional level), thereby acted as a broker between competing and vigorously articulated views. The *Deutsche AIDS-Hilfe*, advocating a combination of health education and intervention at community level, had been brought into being partly as a political counterweight to the Bavarian CSU, which was demanding that health education be backed by legal repression. In this context health education functioned to provide the lowest common denominator of prevention.

The primary contrast between the two countries in respect of AIDS is systemic, being linked to differences in political and health policy structure. Nevertheless, both countries developed a liberal response based on health education and voluntary testing. The means by which these responses were produced, however, were different. Similar policy outcomes therefore can be brought about by different processes and to resolve quite different political problems.

The periodization of policy responses is indicative, of course, of change and process in policy-making. Along the way it has been possible to identify the role of significant non-governmental ASOs in both countries (the Terrence Higgins

Trust and the *Deutsche AIDS-Hilfe*) and differences in their relative profiles. What might a more detailed history reveal about their place in this process?

The Voluntary Sector: Germany

In March 1985 an informal meeting was set up in Düsseldorf by the Federal Centre for Health Education and the Federal Health Office between themselves, federal and regional health officials, clinicians, sexologists and representatives of the *AIDS-Hilfen* to explore possibilities of cooperation over AIDS. At more or less the same time, significant developments were taking place in Berlin; Berlin's Senator for Health and Social Affairs was then Ulf Fink, who belongs to the liberal wing of the CDU and is something of a social policy ideologue. A reorientation of CDU health policy was taking place in this period, during which self-help was discussed at length. In this context Fink had set up a special budget at the senate in Berlin to sponsor local self-help activity in social policy (known as the '*Selbsthilfetopf*'). This was intended to promote speedy and flexible responses to social issues (Fink, 1987).

Furthermore, partly as a result of the size and strength of the gay community in Berlin, the *AIDS-Hilfe* movement was strongest there. It was the *Berliner AIDS-Hilfe* which was restructured to create the two separate agencies *Berliner AIDS-Hilfe* and *Deutsche AIDS-Hilfe*. Berlin, then, saw the conjunction of a new strand of government thinking on health policy, a large and well politicized gay community, and the emergence of AIDS. The relationship between these is perhaps coincidental, but in retrospect it can be seen to have had wide implications. At the very least, AIDS self-help groups represented a field of opportunity for reformist policy-making.

The years 1985–86 saw a *Gründerboom* of AIDS groups in provincial towns (Canaris, 1988; Wübker, 1988). Following discussions in Cologne, the *Deutsche AIDS-Hilfe* (DAH) was founded in Berlin in December 1985 to function as a national networking body. Beyond the necessity of coordinating information and advice provided by different local groups, a need had arisen for the construction of a national lobby and institutional conduit for available federal funds. The formation of the *Deutsche AIDS-Hilfe* was encouraged by and financed through the Federal Centre for Health Education, which was then looking for a correspondent non-governmental policy carrier or partner. The creation of the DAH marked the emergence, therefore, of AIDS self-help onto the national policy stage. Its budget, supplied from federal sources, grew rapidly from DM300,000 in 1985 to 2 million in 1986 and 7 million 1987. This funding, it should be noted, was provided solely for a national networking function; local groups were and are financed by their respective regional states and municipalities.

The *Deutsche AIDS-Hilfe* also has a regional tier. The AH *Landesverband NRW* (a state-wide association of *AIDS-Hilfen* in Nordrhein-Westfalen), for example, was formed in 1987 with twin aims: the exchange of opinion and experience between its member organizations (thirty-two by 1990, one-third of all *AIDS-Hilfen* in the country), and political lobbying, crucial to obtaining funding at the regional state level. The success of AH coordination has been the attainment of a level of independent networking unmatched in any other welfare issue, and this is directly attributable to the extent of federal resourcing it has acquired; *AIDS-Hilfe* networking has been facilitated as much by money from above, as it had been painstakingly constructed from below.

Governing the German Voluntary Sector

Canaris (1988), writing as a former Director of the Federal Centre for Health Education, was clearly impressed by the speed and extent of the establishment of the *Deutsche AIDS-Hilfe* in German health policy, describing the political emergence of the *AIDS-Hilfen* as being testament to the effectiveness of its political lobbying. The *Deutsche AIDS-Hilfe* now holds a seemingly natural and permanent membership of expert hearings and advisory bodies (Wübker, 1988). This has been achieved, moreover, despite the fragmentary, decentralized state of the West German gay movement.

In retrospect, however, the overriding feature of the period is the success of the federal government in imposing its own conception of a division of competence in the AIDS field between the DAH and federal agencies. The basis for this was established in 1985 in Cologne, according to which the DAH was accorded institutional and policy competence for prevention work with groups at risk, meaning, at that stage, with gay men (Canaris, 1988; see also *Deutsche AIDS-Hilfe*, 1989). Responsibility for the provision of general information and education on AIDS continued to rest with the Federal Centre for Health Education. The drawing of a political line between such closely related spheres of activity inevitably proved to be a source of tension. As Federal Minister of Health Rita Süßmuth put it, 'Many *AIDS-Hilfen* don't agree with me on this point. Nevertheless, I think it is right; it's just that the boundaries mustn't become too strict. . . . What we need is sensitive cooperation between statutory and voluntary organisations' (Süßmuth, 1987, pp. 77, 101; author's translation). In turn, the political impact of the introduction of the AIDS Coordination Unit at the Federal Ministry in late 1987 was felt more keenly by the *Deutsche AIDS-Hilfe* than by the Federal Centre for Health Education. DAH budgets, which run through the Centre, were now more tightly controlled by the ministry.

The period 1988–89 saw the emergence of drug users as a central interest in HIV and AIDS prevention. A policy conflict emerged between those advocating harm reduction, involving opiate substitution, and traditional agencies and institutions committed to abstention. The *Deutsche AIDS-Hilfe*, rather than drugs agencies, was the catalyst of a new drugs policy arguing for substitution and harm reduction rather than therapy, developing its recommendations in tandem with the sponsorship of drug user self-help.[11] Even though many of the provincial *AIDS-Hilfen* were born of drugs work, the DAH drug-related budget of DM2.1 million was cut back to DM200,000 in 1988–89. In part, these developments suggest an attempt by government and the established social service interest to manoeuvre *AIDS-Hilfe* back into its 'classical' form (Runze, 1988), that of gay self-help.

The Voluntary Sector: The UK

The Terrence Higgins Trust (THT) has led AIDS work in the voluntary sector in London and, in effect, in the UK, as can be inferred from the capital bias of

British AIDS epidemiology and politics. The Trust was the first ASO in the UK and was for some time de facto the sector's national leader.

The early activity of the THT centred on the production and circulation of AIDS information leaflets; its initial funding came entirely from the gay community. The Trust opened a telephone helpline in February 1984 and began a process of government lobbying over AIDS. It slowly gained in public and political legitimacy during 1983–84, its status enhanced by the formal involvement of London-based specialists in genito-urinary medicine. The Trust was awarded its first government grant of £35,000 in September 1985, and a further £100,000 in mid-1986. For individuals seeking advice and help in relation to AIDS there was, until 1986 and apart from the Terrence Higgins Trust, 'no one else to turn to' (Schramm-Evans, 1990).

The collapse of the Trust's accounting system in the summer of 1987 brought a spate of resignations. Further central funding was delayed by the UK general election in June 1987, and the £330,000 which came subsequently was little more than half that requested. By this time the Department of Health (through the HEA) was itself moving into the same areas, such as leaflet production and distribution, for which it had previously sponsored the Terrence Higgins Trust. Equally, other local groups were beginning to establish themselves, often with THT support. The Trust's uniqueness, seen originally as the source of its power, was being undermined (Schramm-Evans, 1990).

Other AIDS agencies began to emerge up and down the country in 1984–85. At what now can be seen to have been a crucial moment, the THT, in the absence of substantial or official resourcing, decided not to develop a federated national network. It was felt that distance management would be difficult without either a powerful, well-funded centre or clearly defined aims. There was a feeling, too, that local issues required a local response. Beyond that, the Trust was (or had been made to feel) sufficiently cautious about its own activity not to take on responsibility for the actions of others.[12] A member of THT's Review Committee has described the work of the Trust as *providing* direct services for greater London, and *sharing* information and training both nation-wide and world-wide (Gorna, 1990).

This strategy meant that there has emerged no coordinated response to HIV/AIDS in the British voluntary sector. As one experienced voluntary sector AIDS worker put it, 'there is a tendency . . . for the charismatic and therefore for a fractured and splintered response.' There is now a proliferation of organizations in the UK 'beyond the bounds of what is sensible or rational'. Other voluntary sector agencies with a national remit now include those concerned primarily with education, information and research; with lobbying and service delivery; and with fundraising and distribution. The Terrence Higgins Trust had become 'merely the first and still largest of a growing number of voluntary-based AIDS charities throughout the country' (Schramm-Evans, 1990).

Other UK AIDS Organizations

In what was understood as an attempt to 'straighten things out', the UK AIDS Foundation, modelled on the American AMFAR, was set up in 1985 to bring together medical research, clinicians, political parties and the voluntary sector.

This was to constitute a more coherent and cohesive, yet still broadly based AIDS lobby. The attempt, however, quickly failed as the new body disintegrated in political acrimony and disarray.[13] Two groupings emerged during post-UKAF discussion: a pro-medical one, which had access to the Department of Health but understood little of voluntary sector organizations, and a pro-voluntary one, which sought to represent a voluntary sector which was then timid, unsure and over-stretched. The first group ultimately became the National AIDS Trust (NAT); the other, articulating the particular interest of those based outside London, formed the much weaker Network of Voluntary Organisations in HIV/AIDS (NOVOAH).

The establishment of the National AIDS Trust was announced by the Secretary of State for Social Services on 5 May 1987. It reflected a then much-favoured partnership between government and British private enterprise: it was to be chaired by Austin Bide, President of Glaxo Holdings; its fund-raising subcommittee was to be chaired by Robert Maxwell, owner of the Mirror Group. Government funding was set at £500,000 and was initially matched by the private sector; corporate funding then fell to £80,000 in 1989. The work of the National AIDS Trust has evolved into the provision of management training and consultancy for voluntary sector ASOs, and has also focused on what it has identified as the priority areas of housing and prisons. The National AIDS Trust has met with some criticism from voluntary sector agencies in the field.

Important in the formation of the National AIDS Trust was the implicit refusal by government to recognize the potential of existing and well-established bodies (such as the Terrence Higgins Trust) to fulfil the voluntary sector ASO coordinating function. There is also a suggestion that the intention has been to carry AIDS work into what the NAT's Director has described as the 'traditional' voluntary sector (Jay, 1990), if not to transfer its institutional focus altogether. In terms of AIDS politics in the UK, the National AIDS Trust represented a counterweight to the gay lobby.

Governing the UK Voluntary Sector

The Terrence Higgins Trust itself achieved a high profile in the national AIDS policy-making arena during 1985–86, some of its members making significant inputs into the Expert Advisory Group on AIDS formed at the DoH in January 1985. At the level of service delivery, internal discussions took place in the THT in mid-1986 as to whether the Trust was doing something that properly should have been done by the state; THT 'home care', for example, might be regarded as a statutory social service responsibility. In 1986 the reality of the situation was that the state simply wasn't providing services. Since then, social service provision in relation to AIDS has been expanded, while 'care in the community' has become the order of the day. This is to say that the THT, perhaps the flagship of the AIDS-specific voluntary sector, has found itself in the position of having to respond to changes in the statutory sector. In the context of current reform of the NHS, the Terrence Higgins Trust is likely to become a contract supplier of specialist services to local and health authorities, the basis of its activity fundamentally changed.

From 1991, under the impact of health service reform, there will be no further provision for the direct funding of voluntary sector health care by central government

(Section 64 funding); voluntary organizations will be asked to apply to local statutory bodies. For the THT, this will mean that one application to the DoH will be replaced by applications to thirty-three London Boroughs, thirty-one District Health Authorities, four Regional Health Authorities and the HEA.[14] This development has at least three implications: the investment of scant resources simply in obtaining further resources will be demanded by a process of increased bureaucratic complexity; the local voluntary sector will be more closely regulated by statutory bodies with whom it is often in direct competition; and national networking is even more likely to be inhibited by the eclipse of national level funding.

Discussion

Many of the common problems of AIDS service organizations, such as professionalization and bureaucratization, resulting in an increasing distance from the communities in which they were born, and the limitations placed on their activity which come with government funding, are not new to the voluntary sector. They belong, perhaps, to the typical 'organizational career' (cf. Evers, 1990) of the non-profit and non-governmental welfare agency.[15] What is of interest here is their relationship to their external political and organizational environments. What, then, are the significant differences in this regard between Britain and Germany?

First, there is an interesting structural contrast between German federated coherence and British virtual incoherence, which can be described as both centralized and atomized at one and same time. This pattern subverts our standard images of health policy-making in the respective countries.

Second, there is the federal funding of the German *Deutsche AIDS-Hilfe* as early as 1985, while the British government delayed its investment until the formation of the National AIDS Trust in 1987. Third, if we examine the politicization of AIDS in the period 1985–86 and its subsequent depoliticization in the period 1986–87, we can see a gradual shift in policy-making style from the informal to the formal. In the period of informal policy development, the German state quickly looked to establish the *AIDS-Hilfen* as a partner in policy-making; the UK state delayed policy production until the statutory sector (the NHS) and, to a lesser extent, the traditional voluntary sector, were able to reassert themselves.

It is at this point that the 'organizational careers' of respective ASOs diverge. The *Deutsche AIDS-Hilfe* has stabilized in the context of what Evers (1990) characterizes as a form of 'social contract'; its functional competence has been defined (the provision of information and services to those directly affected by AIDS) and its funding sustained. It might well be that the *AIDS-Hilfen* will settle into the status of a conventional German welfare *Verband*. The Terrence Higgins Trust, on the other hand, in the wake of National Health Service Reform introducing an internal market system, seems to have been relegated to subcontractor status. Where the German state may be said to have entered into a contractual relationship with its major ASO, the relationship between the UK state and a set of weakened ASOs is better described as one of exploitation. As one UK AIDS worker observed, the statutory sector, rather than working with it, expects to take *from* the voluntary sector. The German government is much more ready to work *with* the non-profit sector.

The German government, it has been argued, used the *AIDS-Hilfen* to gain a foothold in local health politics. The federal state has no capacity for service delivery in health and welfare; hospital provision is the responsibility of the regional state. By constitutional law (the *Grundgesetz*) government responsibility for public health is accorded to the regional states; in some states this has been devolved to the municipalities. The federal government, therefore, may not interfere in public health policy other than by providing short-term 'model' funding. Struggling elsewhere for the political authority to impose cost containment on the health sector, its distributive measures in respect of AIDS, its financing of the *Modellprogramme* and its sponsorship of the DAH gave the federal government leverage at the lowest and most local level of health administration as it circumvented, albeit temporarily, constitutionally given hierarchies (Czada and Friedrich-Czada, 1990). For the British government, funding options for AIDS work were broader, yet perhaps easier and more straightforward. It could choose among local authorities, the voluntary sector and the local subunit of the NHS, the District Health Authority. Disliking local authorities and unhappy with the face of the voluntary sector with which it was presented, central government flushed the large part of AIDS funding through the NHS (see Beardshaw, 1989; Beardshaw, Hunter and Taylor, 1990). The NHS, of course, represented not only a local statutory funding option unavailable to the Germans, but also a conduit of medical, influence on British government policy.

German public health policy may be seen as a product of conflict, negotiation and the interplay of competences between Bund and Länder. German Federalism contributed to the production of policy conflict over AIDS in two ways: by allowing an opportunity for political bidding by a relatively small party with a strong local power base (the Bavarian CSU) and by enabling access for pressure groups such as the *AIDS-Hilfen* (c.f. Katzenstein, 1987). By increasing the number of locations of state power, where regional and municipal government enjoy both policy autonomy and independent financial resource, federalism increases the range of political opportunity for non-established groups. There is a clear contrast here with the centralizing thrust of Thatcherite policy in the UK (Gamble, 1988) and its unwillingness to delegate policy competences to institutions and agencies other than those under its direct influence. To put this a slightly different way, Czada and Friedrich-Czada (1990) suggest that unitary political systems tend to have dealt with AIDS by developing programmes within their existing administrative structures, while those with fragmented health policy systems take more direct account of those to whom policy is addressed. Symbolic policy-making is more difficult in federal systems, owing to the existence of more centres of political accountability.

The development of the third sector response to AIDS is shaped, of course, by the structure of the pro-existing policy arena to which the issue has been assigned. AIDS in the UK has been defined as a health, that is, a medical issue. The UK health policy arena is dominated by the National Health Service which, in its reorganizations of 1974 and 1982 and in subsequent reviews, has gradually assumed responsibility for prevention, health promotion and public health. German health policy in respect of prevention, however, is without a major player or established interest. Germany does, though, have a well developed third sector in welfare, into which the self-help movement, and especially those groups with a health-related function, is making considerable inroads (Trojan, Halves and Wetendorf, 1986).

Conclusions

AIDS policy seems to correlate with no single variable in Type 1 countries. It does not correlate with parties in government, or with political systems (Czada and Friedrich-Czada, 1990). Policy responses to AIDS seem instead to be unusually idiosyncratic, shaped by particular combinations of tradition, ideology, organizational forms and varying strengths of established interest, of policy-making style and current political intent. Which of these influences on AIDS policy-making is strongest?

Fox, Day and Klein (1989), discussing the US, British and Swedish cases, write of the 'power of professionalism' in determining AIDS policies, which they describe as 'evidence of the authority that medical, scientific and public health professionals have acquired during this century.' This is felt by some to overplay the degree of influence held by medical and scientific actors, and to ignore or even undermine the significant input into AIDS policy-making made by those directly affected, particularly in the early stages of policy formulation (Strong and Berridge, 1990).

The reverse side of the Fox, Day and Klein argument has been examined in this chapter, to place criticism of it in perspective. It is suggested that we may begin to explain policy responses to AIDS, in a comparative context, by looking at the often widely varying health and social policy arenas in which they have been produced. This means, for example, that two sets of relationships warrant further attention: that between the state and the health sector, and that between statutory and voluntary agencies.

Notes

1 There are some examples in the UK literature — see, for example, Berridge and Strong (1990), Day and Klein (1989), Schramm-Evans (1990), Street (1988), Strong and Berridge (1990) and Weeks (1989) — but few on Germany. One of these is in English (Pollak, 1990) and one in German (Canaris, 1988). Rühmann (1985) gives early impressions, and Gerhardt (1988) is also valuable. The German literature, perhaps predictably, is much more concerned with aspects of law than with policy-making.

2 Fox, Day and Klein (1989) discuss the US, Britain and Sweden, and there is a valuable comparative element in Czada and Friedrich-Czada (1990). Moerkerk and Aggleton (1990) are among the very few to have attempted a typology of AIDS prevention strategies in Europe. They concentrate, however, as they acknowledge, on what they describe as 'official' policy and take little account of the activity of non-governmental organizations (NGOs).

3 For material on Sweden, the third member of Moerkerk and Aggleton's 'political' category, see Gould (1988), Henriksson (1988), Rosenbrock (1988) and Fox, Day and Klein (1989).

4 The English 'voluntary' can be a confusing and unsatisfactory term. It is used here to refer to welfare agencies which are both non-governmental or non-statutory, and non-profit-making. Similarly, the denotation 'AIDS service organization' (ASO), while current in the comparative literature, should not be understood to exclude the lobbying and representative function of many, if not most, of them.

5 AIDS policy in Germany is currently facing the new challenge set by unification with the GDR. This constitutes a general challenge to political, economic and

social systems within which AIDS, in contrast to abortion but in common with much of the social policy field, has attracted no particular attention. As in the economic sphere, the pattern of social policy development seems, at the end of 1990, to be one of colonization of East by West. Policy responsibility for AIDS can be expected to be carried, as in the West German model, by the newly formed East German *Länder* and, within them, the municipalities. Given the overwhelming statism of political and administrative culture, prospects for ASOs may be unfavourable in the short to medium term. The problem is likely to be less in the foundation of groups, of which there seem to be many (see Süß, 1990) than in relationships with an administrating bureaucracy acknowledged to be inexperienced in the support of non-state initiatives (Sönnichsen, 1990).

6 *Koalitionsvereinbarung zwischen CDU/CSU und FDP vom März 1987*, repr. BMJFFG (1990). For further information on the purpose and content of the *Modellprogramme*, see BMJFFG (1990).

7 *Gesundheitsministerkonferenz (GMK), Sondersitzung*, 27 March 1987.

8 The Bavarian policy catalogue included provision for forcible testing for HIV on suspicion on involvement in sex work or injecting drug use, and the criminalization of intentional or negligent transmission of HIV. Settlement in Bavaria was made conditional on proof of HIV-antibody negative status (cf. *Bekanntmachung des Bayerischen Staatsministeriums des Innern vom 19, 5, 1987 zum Vollzug des Seuchenrechts, des Auslanderrechts und des Polizeirechts*, repr. AIFO 2 (6).

9 For an introductory account of the policy and practice of the *AIDS-Hilfe*, see Hopfner and Beißwenger (1988) and Deutsche AIDS-Hilfe (1989).

10 For further analysis of local AIDS policy in the UK, see Pye, Kapila, Buckley and Cunningham (1989) and Beardshaw, Hunter and Taylor (1990).

11 The self-help group *Junkies, Ex-user and Substituierte* (JES) was formed under the auspices of the DAH in the summer of 1989. The *Junkie Bund Koln* was set up in May 1990.

12 Much of AIDS policy-making in the UK took place in a climate of anti-homosexual repression, centred on the passage through parliament of the Local Government Act (1988). Clause 28 of the Act prohibited local authorities from 'promoting homosexuality by teaching or by publishing material'.

13 Immediately prior to the first public meeting of the UKAF, chair Gerald Vaughan, briefly a Conservative health minister, was quoted in the press as having said that African students entering the UK should be tested for HIV. This comment was clearly unacceptable to the other members of the Foundation, which then collapsed as they withdrew their support.

14 Parliamentary AIDS Digest 4, December 1989.

15 For introductory reviews of voluntary sector research, see Anheier (1990) and Evers (1990).

References

ANHEIER, H. (1990) 'Zur internationalen Forschung über den Nonprofit Sector: Themen und Ansätze', *Journal für Socialforschung*, 30, 2, pp. 163–80.

BEARDSHAW, V. (1989) 'Blunted Weapons', *New Statesman and Society*, 1 December, pp. 24–5.

BEARDSHAW, V., HUNTER, D.J. and TAYLOR, R.C.R. (1990) *Local AIDS Policies. Planning and Policy Development for Health Promotion*, AIDS Programme Paper 6, London, HEA.

BERRIDGE, V. and STRONG, P. (1990) 'AIDS Policies in the UK: A Preliminary Analysis', in E. FEE and D. FOX (Eds), *AIDS: Contemporary History*, Princeton, N.J., Princeton University Press.

BMJFFG (Bundesministerium für Jugend, Familie, Frauen und Gesundheit) (1990) *Aidsbekämpfung in der Bundesrepublik Deutschland*, Bonn, BMJFFG.

BUNIKOWSKI, R., SCHWARTLÄNDER, B., KOCH, M.A. and L'ÂGE STEHR, J. (1989) 'Das Zentrale AIDS-Fallregister: Bericht über die bis 31, Dezember 1988 gemeldeten AIDS-Fälle', AIDS-Forschung (AIFO) 3.

CANARIS, U. (1988) 'Gesundheitpolitische Aspekte im Zusammenhang mit AIDS', in J. KORPORAL and H. MALOUSCHEK (Hg.), *Leben mit AIDS — mit AIDS leben*, Hamburg, EBV.

CZADA, R. and FRIEDRICH-CZADA, H. (1990) 'AIDS als politisches Konfliktfeld und Verwaltungsproblem', in R. ROSENBROCK and A. SALMEN (Hg.), *AIDS-Prävention*, Berlin, Rainer Bohn Verlag.

DAY, P. and KLEIN, R. (1989) 'Interpreting the Unexpected: The Case of AIDS Policy Making in Britain', *Journal of Public Policy*, 9, 3, pp. 337–53.

DEUTSCHE AIDS-HILFE (1987) Memorandum. Leben mit AIDS-Bestandsaufname und Perspektiven der AIDS-Bekämpfung in der Bundesrepublik Deutschland, Berlin, Deutsche AIDS-Hilfe.

DEUTSCHE AIDS-HILFE (1989) *The Concept of Prevention of the Deutsche AIDS-Hilfe*, Berlin, Deutsche AIDS-Hilfe.

EVERS, A. (1990) 'Im intermediären Bereich — soziale Träger und Projekte zwischen Haushalt, Staat und Markt', *Journal für Sozialforschung*, 30, 2, pp. 189–210.

FINK, U. (1987) 'AIDS geht jeden an', in Senator für Gesundheit und Soziales (Berlin) *AIDS geht jeden an. Ergebnisse der internationalen AIDS-Tagung im November 1986 in Berlin*, Berlin, Kulturbuch-Verlag.

FOX, D., DAY, P. and KLEIN, R. (1989) 'The Power of Professionalism: AIDS in Britain, Sweden and the United States', *Daedalus*, 118, pp. 93–112.

FRANZKOWIAK, P. (1989) 'AIDS-Prävention bei Jugendlichen, Konzeptionelle Überlegungen und erste Praxiserfahrungen aus einem Modellprogramm in Nordrhein-Westfalen', *Prävention*, 12, 3, pp. 67–71.

GAMBLE, A. (1988) *The Free Economy and the Strong State*, London, Macmillan.

GERHARDT, U. (1988) 'Zur Effektivität der konkurrierenden Programme der AIDS-Kontrolle. Medizinsoziologische Überlegungen', in B. SHÜNEMANN and G. PFEIFFER (Hg.), *Die Rechtsprobleme von AIDS*, Baden-Baden, Nomos Verlagsgesellschaft.

GORNA, R. (1990) *The Trust Newsletter*, Terrence Higgins Trust, January.

GOULD, A. (1988) *Conflict and Control in Welfare Policy: The Swedish Experience*, Harlow, Longman.

HACHMANN, M., LANGEMANN, U. und BARGSTEDT, P. (1990) *AIDS-Prävention an Schulen: Zwischenbilanz des Berliner Schoolworker-Programms*, Berlin, Arbeitsgruppe AIDS der Senatsverwaltung für Gesundheit und Soziales im Landesinstitut für Tropenmedizin.

HENRIKSSON, B. (1988) *Social Democracy or Societal Control: A Critical Analysis of Swedish AIDS Policy*, Berlin, Wissenschaftszentrum Berlin, WZB papers, 88–205.

HÖPFNER, C. and BEIβWENGER, H-D (1988) 'Konzepte, Strategien und Arbeitsweisen der Aids-Hilfe', in V. SIGUSCH and S. FLIEGEL (Hg.), *AIDS, Ergebnisse des Kongresses fur klinische Psychologie und Psychotherapie, Berlin 1988*, Tübingen, Deutsche Gesellschaft fur Verhaltenstherapie, Tübingen, Reihe 9.

JAY, M. (1990) *AIDS Dialogue 6*, June, 6.

KATZENSTEIN, P.J. (1987) *Policy and Politics in West Germany: The Growth of a Semisovereign State*, Philadelphia, Penn., Temple University Press.

MOERKERK, H. and AGGLETON, P. (1990) 'AIDS Prevention Strategies in Europe: A Comparison and Critical Analysis', in P. AGGLETON, P. DAVIES, and G. HART (Eds), *AIDS: Individual, Cultural and Policy Dimensions*, Lewes, Falmer Press.

POLLAK, M. (1990) 'AIDS in West Germany: Co-ordinating Policy in a Federal System', in B.A. MISZTAL and D. MOSS (Eds), *Action on AIDS: National Policies in Comparative Perspective*, New York, Greenwood.

PYE, M., KAPILA, M. BUCKLEY, G. and CUNNINGHAM, D. (1989) (Eds), *Responding to the AIDS Challenge: A Comparative Study of Local AIDS Programmes in the United Kingdom*, Harlow, Longman/HEA.

ROSENBROCK, R. (1988) *AIDS in Sweden*, Berlin, Wissenschaftszentrum Berlin, WZB papers, 88–205.

RÜHMANN, F. (1985) *AIDS: Eine Krankheit und ihre Folgen*, Frankfurt, Campus.

RUNZE, D. (1988) interviewed in dgsp-rundbrief, *Deutsche Gesellschaft für soziale Psychiatrie, Koln*, 41, June.

SCHRAMM-EVANS, Z. (1990) 'Responses to AIDS: 1986–1987', in P. AGGLETON, P. DAVIES, and G. HART (Eds), *AIDS: Individual, Cultural and Policy Dimensions*, Lewes, Falmer Press.

SÖNNICHSEN, N. (1990) 'AIDS in der DDR: Strategie mit neuer Aktualität', *AIFO*, 5, 1.

STREET, J. (1988) 'British Government Policy on AIDS: Learning Not to Die of Ignorance', *Parliamentary Affairs*, 41, 4, pp. 490–507.

STRONG, P. and BERRIDGE, V. (1990) 'No One Knew Anything: Some Issues in British AIDS Policy', in P. AGGLETON, P. DAVIES, and G. HART (Eds), *AIDS: Individual, Cultural and Policy Dimensions*, Lewes, Falmer Press.

SÜβ, P. (1990) 'AIDS-Hilfen in der DDR. Nichts Genaues weiβ man nicht', *DAH Aktuell*, April/Mai.

SÜβMUTH, R. (1987) *Wege aus der Angst*, Hamburg, Hoffman und Campe Verlag.

TROJAN, A., HALVES, E. and WETENDORF, H.-W. (1986) 'Self-help Groups and Consumer Participation: A Look at the German Health Care Self-help Movement', *Journal of Voluntary Action Research*, 15, 2, pp. 14–23.

WEEKS, J. (1989) 'AIDS: The Intellectual Agenda', in P. AGGLETON, P. DAVIES and G. HART (Eds), *AIDS: Social Representations, Social Practices*, Lewes, Falmer Press.

WÜBKER, A. (1988) *Struktur und Bedeutung der AIDS-Hilfeorganisationen in der Bundesrepublik Deutschland*, Berlin, Deutsche AIDS-Hilfe, AIDS-Forum DAH.

5   Female Prostitution and AIDS: The Realities of Social Exclusion

Graham Scambler and Rebecca Graham-Smith

Since it has become more widely realized that HIV infection could be heterosexually transmitted, renewed attention has been paid to the role and patterns of behaviour of women sex workers. In the work of some commentators and policy-makers in the mid-1980s, women in the sex industry were promptly, and with numerous historical precedents, cast as putative vectors of disease. In the first part of this chapter we briefly draw on this material to reflect both on how women sex workers continue to be objects of vilification, regarded as morally and causally responsible for the spread of sexually transmitted diseases (STDs), including AIDS; and on how this very process of vilification enhances the vulnerability to infection of the women themselves, their clients and others in the wider community. We then define and assess the potential of *operational*, *political* and *structural* changes to empower women sex workers better to safeguard their own health, a process of special salience in the context of HIV/AIDS. The roles and relationships of sex workers, prostitute groups and the women's movement will also be addressed as part of a consideration of likely agencies of change.

Women Sex Workers and AIDS

Many women sex workers in the mid-1980s took exception to assertions or insinuations that they had a high probability of becoming infected with HIV, that they might infect other 'normal' people, and that they might need to be monitored and put under some stricter form of surveillance. Some, and with some cause, experienced contemporary epidemiological research focusing on the prevalence of HIV infection and types of sexual behaviour among sex workers as intrusive, a form of surveillance in its own right. What this same research suggested by the late 1980s, however, was that fewer women sex workers than some had first supposed were HIV seropositive. One of the first longitudinal studies in London, for example, found that only three out of 187 women sex workers attending a clinic and tested for HIV were positive for HIV antibodies (Day *et al.*, 1988). Significantly, two of these three were injecting drug users and the third had almost certainly been infected by a boyfriend, who was also found to be HIV seropositive.

Epidemiological and, increasingly, sociological research on women sex workers and HIV/AIDS now presents a complex picture (Plant, 1990). Rather than review all the relevant studies here (see Graham-Smith and Scambler 1991), we will identify a number of themes in current research and debate which are, we believe, consonant with empirical findings. First, as both conventional historical treatises and polemical feminist tracts (e.g., Wells, 1982) testify, women sex workers have been routinely used and abused for centuries under the auspices of patriarchal normative and legal systems. A double standard of sexual morality has persisted, with the use of sex workers being as forgivable in a man as being one is unforgivable in a woman (McIntosh, 1981). With all due allowance for what Elias (1978) has termed 'the civilizing process' in the West, this remains true in contemporary Britain. If prostitution per se is not actually illegal, women engaged in sex work continue to be regarded as social outcasts, and the police and courts are intermittently mobilized to pursue and harrass them, especially if they are conspicuous as street workers. The Sexual Offences Act of 1956, aimed at male profiteers, and the Sexual Offences Act of 1985, criminalizing male kerb crawling, are largely unenforceable against men and, in their effect, further disadvantage women at work (Scambler *et al.*, 1990). In Britain today women sex workers remain as unacceptable as people or citizens as they are in demand as providers of sexual services.

Second, the social unacceptability of women sex workers has long made them ready targets in the event of outbreaks, or perceived outbreaks, of STDs. One of the best documented British illustrations of this occurred when, as a result of public concern at the high prevalence of venereal disease among troops, the Contagious Diseases Acts of 1864, 1866 and 1869 were passed (Walkowitz, 1980). Even making allowance for the fact that venereal disease was at the time medically defined as transmitted only by women, it is remarkable that no attempts were made to restrain men from placing themselves at risk; instead, the Acts brought the police and judiciary into play to force women sex workers into medical quarantine. Pateman (1988, p. 196) quotes from the Report of a Royal Commission into the Acts, which state that 'there is no comparison to be made between prostitutes and the men who consort with them. With the one sex, the offence is committed as a matter of gain; with the other, it is an irregular indulgence of a natural impulse.' This episode and others provide historical precedents for affording the woman worker the pre-eminent and demeaning status of vector of disease.

Although it is now widely acknowledged, at least in Britain, that mandatory schemes for screening, testing or incarcerating women sex workers as a means of preventing HIV/AIDS would drive them (further) underground, and thus prove counter-productive (Morgan Thomas *et al.*, 1989), there is little doubt that the initial attempts to research and influence sex workers' behaviour in the mid-1980s were more informed by concern about HIV transmission into the wider population than about the vulnerability of women sex workers themselves.

Third, sex work is not in itself a risk factor for HIV infection; rather, certain behaviours and circumstances associated with it may enhance a woman's vulnerability to infection. The two 'vulnerability factors' that stand out are injecting drug use (IDU) and unprotected sex. Rates of injecting drug use among women sex workers vary, often by locality. Where rates are high, as in Edinburgh where about 20 per cent of women sex workers inject, rates of HIV infection may be enhanced. From a 'snowball' sample of 103 working women in Edinburgh, twelve of those who both reported having had an HIV antibody test and were able or willing to reveal the results were seropositive. Of these twelve, nine were injecting drug users, one said that her regular partner was an HIV seropositive injecting drug user, and two told of former boyfriends known to be seropositive (Morgan Thomas *et al.*, 1989). The authors of a study of women sex workers working on the streets in Glasgow have recently reported that an alarming 59 per cent of them were injecting drug users (McKeganey *et al.*, 1990). While the sharing of needles or 'works' is generally assumed to account for infection among injecting drug using sex workers, women are also at risk from male-to-female sexual transmission (Rosenberg and Weiner, 1988).

Studies have consistently shown high, and rising, condom use with commercial sexual contacts. Rates of use are often dramatically lower, however, with boyfriends. Day and Ward (1990) have suggested that this marked difference in sexual behaviour is of deep symbolic significance. Condoms, it appears, are as important as symbolic barriers between women sex workers and their clients as their absence is important for continuing intimacy with their boyfriends. But boyfriends too can be injecting drug users and/or be having unsafe sex outside their primary relationship. Day and her colleagues (1987) see a possible tension here since 'a paradoxical situation could arise in which women prostitutes become HIV infected from their boyfriends but their clients remain protected through universal condom use.'

Suspending any qualms about the motivation that may underpin research on women sex workers, evidence of their vulnerability to HIV infection, notably through injecting drug use and unprotected sex, is clear. It has also become increasingly apparent that many women sex workers have health needs in general as well as in relation to STDs, including HIV/AIDS, which are not being met. The principal cause would seem to be lack of access to appropriate and user-friendly services. Moreover, when, as sometimes occurs, good quality primary or secondary care is available, the route to it often appears hazardous or circuitous. Even well-informed and committed outreach workers who regard the health of women sex workers as important in its own right rather than merely for containing HIV disease have found it immensely hard to make headway (Graham-Smith and Scambler, 1991).

Ending Social Exclusion: Recommendations for Change

Social norms condemning sex work, articulated in law and enforced through police and court activity, constitute the major impediment to safeguarding the health of women in the sex industry. By defining and legitimating the harassment of women as deviants and misfits, they open a gap between working women and the health and related services which cannot easily be bridged. There is evidence of this in the testimonies of health workers in STD clinics and outreach programmes, as well as in almost all recent studies of sex work in relation to HIV infection.

Two categories of problem will be discussed here. One *specific* problem relates to the manner in which women sex workers are policed. McLeod (1982;

p. 109) has shown how in Birmingham the police 'do not lack initiative or inventiveness extending their powers in relation to prostitution.' She cites their use in 1980 of fourteenth century statutes against kerb crawlers, the object being to reduce the numbers of street workers by scaring away potential clients. More common are sporadic and intensive police campaigns to enforce the 1959 Street Offences Act against selected groups of street workers. Kinnell (1989) suggests that such campaigns act to destroy or disrupt the contacts with women that are slowly and painstakingly being established by outreach workers. Police activity *against* street workers routinely undermines health and HIV/AIDS programmes *for* street workers.

Police activity is dysfunctional in other ways. It discourages the dissemination of literature and the distribution of condoms to women and their clients. Many women fear that possessing safer-sex materials developed for sex workers or condoms may be used as evidence in prosecution, or as a basis for police harassment. Clubs or agencies are similarly unwilling to distribute safer-sex pamphlets in case these are later used as evidence in prosecution. The imposition of heavy fines on street workers may force them back to work to raise money; and unsafe sex, which is typically more lucrative, can be another temptation when funds are short.

Second, and perhaps more importantly, a *general* problem is the high level of suspicion and wariness among women sex workers, not just of the police but of all those charged with representing and defending relevant public mores. This extends to the probation, social and health services, and even into the voluntary sector (McLeod, 1982). Over and beyond the possibility of meeting with condescension, chastisement, moral exhortation or pity, women fear the power of 'officials' to complicate, constrain and control their lives. The sense of persecution and injustice is frequently sharp.

Three kinds of change need to be considered: operational, political and structural. *Operational* changes are those which are credible within the existing social and cultural climate of Britain; they offer a challenging but 'negotiable' package of options in relation to appropriate health provision, police activity, and support for women in difficulty or wanting to leave sex work (see Graham-Smith and Scambler, 1991). While important, full implementation of these would almost certainly do little to safeguard further the health and well-being of women sex workers. It would be an exercise in damage limitation.

Political change is more controversial. At its core is the thesis that 'voluntary adult sex work' should be decriminalized. Decriminalization — or 'the abolition of laws and sentences which discriminate against women who work as prostitutes' (McLeod, 1982, p. 119) — has been the subject of campaigns in the USA and Europe since the 1970s. These campaigns have usually been characterized as 'belonging' within the women's movement. Alexander (1988, p. 184) claims that 'there is a growing realization among many feminists that the laws against prostitution, and the stigma imposed on sex work, keep all women from determining their own sexuality.' Moreover, many feminists perceive sex workers, and especially street workers, as a harshly oppressed minority of women.

But decriminalization is not the only political recommendation for change. Other companion measures are to be found in a World Charter produced by the International Committee for Prostitutes' Rights (ICPR) (see Delacoste and Alexander, 1988). These include the enforcement of existing legislation against fraud, coercion, rape, child abuse and so on; the regulation of third parties, the granting of civil rights for women sex workers, and the extension of the taxation and benefits system to them; as well as help and support for women wishing to leave sex work. No claim is made that the implementation of this family of measures would *in itself* guarantee a greatly improved situation for women workers. However, political action on the basis of the World Charter would formally restore the principal rights of citizenship to working women and pave the way for the eventual desegregation of a body of women long excluded from society. Desegregation, in turn, would assist in the removal of barriers between women sex workers and health and companion workers.

Apart from noting that the obvious alternatives to decriminalization, all of them associated with segregation (Darrow, 1984), have done little to safeguard sex workers' health or to counter the spread of STDs, two additional points might be made. First, decriminalization is now in the process of being implemented in the Netherlands, where the sex workers' rights groups, Red Thread, has been particularly active and influential, and where the culture is more liberal than Britain's. Only 'enforced prostitution' is to be illegal, and Venema and Visser (1990, p. 58) are confident that, if cities ensure that individual sex workers are not compelled to register, 'the general health of those in the sex industry will be enhanced.'

The second point is an important qualification to the support for decriminalization offered here. While it has been contended that decriminalization would almost certainly benefit women's health and facilitate HIV/AIDS prevention programmes, it is *not* being asserted either that the probable health return is in itself a sufficient ground for decriminalization or that there are not powerful arguments against decriminalization. The advocacy of decriminalization here is unequivocal, but the full case for it must be made elsewhere. Those feminists who oppose decriminalization as a flawed 'sexual liberalism' understandably fear that it could give additional social legitimacy to the ideology and practice of male dominance in social and sexual relations, currently epitomized in the institution of sex work (Giobbe, 1990). Such a view leads naturally to the desire to 'bring about a situation where the need for sex work is abolished because male-female relations will not be dominated by sexism and material inequality' (McLeod, 1982, p. 69). It is a view, in short, which anticipates the supersession of modern patriarchal capitalism by a new social order (Scambler *et al.*, 1990).

It is apt now to turn to the third kind of recommendation for change, which we have termed *structural*. To oversimplify, just as operational changes are likely to be only minimally effective in the absence of political changes like decriminalization, so changes in the political domain will have a predictably limited impact without concomitant structural changes. Decriminalization, or even the enactment of the ICPR programme as a whole, would not guarantee equality of respect or compassion for women sex workers, nor would it immediately alter their self-perceptions or others' perceptions of them. In the short term more women might perhaps turn to sex work, given that women are not infrequently 'driven or recruited to sex work for want of alternative means to subsist and provide as single parents' (Scambler *et al.*, 1990, p. 269), and that rates of relative poverty are currently increasing rather than decreasing among groups of women like single mothers in Britain (Oppenheim, 1990). In the medium term structural changes to reduce capitalist Britain's class and gender inequalities in public and private domains alike are required to maximize the effectiveness and decriminalization of sex work. In the long term, paradoxically, and with a whiff of what Giddens (1990) has termed 'Utopian realism', structural changes to reduce further or to eliminate such inequalities may render sex work as it has been known hitherto more or less defunct.

The Women's Movement and Sex Worker Representation

The prospects for achieving in Britain the political and structural changes described here are discouraging, even in the long term. What possibilities there are rely for their success on sponsorship by the women's movement. Most contemporary theorists regard the women's movement as an, or even *the*, exemplar of what are termed 'new social movements'. While the discontinuities between the largely class-based old social movements and the new social movements can be exaggerated (Scott, 1990), it is generally accepted that the latter have distinctive qualities. According to Cohen (1985, p. 664), they all raise the theme of the 'self-defence of "society" against the state (and the market economy)'. Habermas (1981) makes the same point when he suggests that, for all their considerable heterogeneity, new social movements are united in their 'resistance to tendencies to colonize the lifeworld'. The more progressive new social movements are engaged in struggles to achieve a democratic civil society. Habermas goes on to define the women's movement as the one current movement which is at the same time progressive, offensive rather than defensive, and committed to universalistic rather than particularistic demands (Scambler, 1987).

According to Eyerman and Jamison (1991, p. 91), the events of the 1960s were pivotal in the development of the new social movements: 'the 1960s opened the space for the later movements to fill with specific meanings'. During the late 1960s and the 1970s the women's movement, like the other new social movements, provided 'a kind of specialization to the rather overextended cosmological ambitions of the 1960s' (*ibid.*). By the late 1980s, however, the women's movement, again in line with others, had 'largely been incorporated into established politics' (*ibid.*), in the guise of academic departments or appointments in women's studies and so on.

Part of Eyerman and Jamison's intention is to bring 'meaning' back into the study of social movements, and they set out to accomplish this using the concepts of *cognitive praxis* and *movement intellectual*. Cognitive praxis, or the production of new knowledge, is defined as the core activity of a social movement. They add:

> a social movement is not one organization or one particular special interest group. It is more like a cognitive territory, a new conceptual space that is filled by a dynamic interaction between different groups and organizations. It is through tensions between different organizations over defining and acting in that conceptual space that the (temporary) identity of a social movement is formed. (Eyerman and Jamison, 1991, p. 55)

A movement intellectual is an individual who participates in the formation of a social movement and, through his or her activities, gives expression to the 'cognitive

identity' of that movement. Over time, an intellectual formed within a movement
may seek legitimacy in more established intellectual havens, like universities or
the media; thus Eyerman and Jamison distinguished between movement and establishment intellectuals.

By utilizing Eyerman and Jamison's cognitive approach to new social movements, we can highlight just two of the multiple 'tensions' within the women's
movement concerning sex workers. The first of these has found expression in the
protracted, continuing and often polarized debate between movement and latterly
established intellectuals on the meaning and significance of pornography. For *radical*
feminists like Dworkin (1981), sexuality and violence are at the core of men's
power over women. She characterizes pornography as 'the graphic depiction of
women as vile whores'. 'The metaphysics of male sexual domination is that women
are whores' (*ibid.*, p. 68). Pornography and prostitution *constitute* violence against
women; both are forms of sexual colonization of women's bodies by men and, as
such, must unequivocally be opposed by all women. For *liberal* feminists on the
other hand, of paramount concern is the individual's freedom to sell, buy or
object to pornography or sexual services; they favour a free market.

No attempt will be made here to examine this debate in detail. It will be
apparent, however, both that advocacy of the decriminalization of sex work is
incompatible with a radical stance; and that, if decriminalization is to occur,
sponsorship elsewhere within the movement will be required. In this sense the
debate between movement and establishment intellectuals has deep practical import. But it is not simply a matter of advocating liberal as opposed to radical
feminism. As Assiter (1991) has shown, the theses advanced by many radicals *and*
liberals share highly contestable 'individualist' foundations. Neither, for example,
can adequately account for the social realities of class, race and big business. Any
shift away from a radical stance within the women's movement, therefore, would
need to be appropriately grounded for decriminalization, even if attained, to benefit
women sex workers more than marginally.

The second tension is between the largely establishment intellectuals within
the women's movement, especially but not exclusively those espousing radical
feminist theories on pornography and prostitution, and those movement intellectuals formed through the emergence of sex worker groups in the USA and
Europe in the 1970s, most of them sex workers or ex-sex workers, and many
of them tending to a more liberal stance (Delacoste and Alexander, 1988). The
tension here is not merely between conflicting theories or stances, but between
insiders and *outsiders*, that is, between women in or from the sex industry (sometimes caricatured by outsiders as men's dupes or victims) and women lacking such
involvement (sometimes caricatured by insiders as 'fucking madonnas'). Although there have been several worthwhile attempts to initiate dialogue between
insiders and outsiders, most notably perhaps the gathering in Ontario documented
by Bell (1987), it will require much time and goodwill if the tension is to be
overcome.

To the extent that the desegregation and restored citizenship of women sex
workers, with their probable health return, are contingent on the support of the
women's movement, tensions like these, and many more — for example, between
movement intellectuals in organized sex worker groups and the sex worker community — will need to be adequately addressed. The kind of political and structural
changes discussed earlier in this chapter certainly require as much.

References

ALEXANDER, P. (1988) 'Prostitution: A Difficult Issue for Feminists', in F. DELACOSTE and P. ALEXANDER (Eds), *Sex Work: Writings by Women in the Sex Industry*, London, Virago Press.

ASSITER, A. (1991) *Pornography, Feminism and the Individual*, London, Pluto Press.

BELL, L. (Ed.) (1987) *Good Girls/Bad Girls: Sex Trade Workers and Feminists Face to Face*, Toronto, The Women's Press.

COHEN, J. (1985) 'Strategy or Identity; New Theoretical Paradigms and Contemporary Social Movements', *Social Research*, 52, pp. 663–716.

DARROW, W. (1984) 'Prostitution and Sexually Transmitted Diseases', in K. HOLMES, P. MARDH, P. SPARLING and P. WIESNER (Eds), *Sexually Transmitted Diseases*, New York, McGraw-Hill.

DAY, S. and WARD, H. (1990) 'The Praed Street Project: A Cohort of Prostitute Women in London', in M. PLANT (Ed.), *AIDS, Drugs and Prostitution*, London, Routledge.

DAY, S., WARD, H., WADSWORTH, J. and HARRIS, J. (1987) 'Attitudes to Barrier Protection among Female Prostitutes in London', Unpublished paper, London, St Mary's Hospital Medical School.

DAY, S., WARD, H. and HARRIS, J. (1988) 'Prostitute Women and Public Health', *British Medical Journal*, 297, p. 1585.

DELACOSTE, F. and ALEXANDER, P. (Eds) (1988) *Sex Work: Writings by Women in the Sex Industry*, London, Virago Press.

DWORKIN, A. (1981) *Pornography: Men Possessing Women*, London, The Women's Press.

ELIAS, N. (1978) *The Civilizing Process: The History of Manners*, Oxford, Blackwell.

EYERMAN, R. and JAMISON, A. (1991) *Social Movements: A Cognitive Approach*, Cambridge, Polity Press.

GIDDENS, A. (1990) *The Consequences of Modernity*, Cambridge, Polity Press.

GIOBBE, E. (1990) 'Confronting the Liberal Lies about Prostitution', in D. LEIDHOLDT and J. RAYMOND (Eds), *The Sexual Liberals and the Attack on Feminism*, Oxford, Pergamon Press.

GRAHAM-SMITH, R. and SCAMBLER, G. (1991) 'Sociological Reflections on Health Care Provision for Women Prostitutes', Unpublished paper.

HABERMAS, J. (1981) 'New Social Movement', *Telos*, 57, pp. 194–205.

KINNELL, H. (1989) 'Prostitutes, Their Clients and Risks of HIV Infection in Birmingham', Occasional paper, Birmingham, Central Birmingham Health Authority, Department of Public Health Medicine.

MCINTOSH, M. (1981) 'Who Needs Prostitutes? The Ideology of Male Sexual Needs', in C. SMART and B. SMART (Eds), *Women, Sexuality and Social Control*, London, Routledge and Kegan Paul.

MCKEGANEY, N., BARNARD, M., BLOOR, M. and LEYLAND, A. (1990) 'Injecting Drug Use and Female Street-working Prostitution in Glasgow', *AIDS*, 4, pp. 1153–5.

MCLEOD, E. (1982) *Working Women: Prostitution Now*, London, Croom Helm.

MORGAN THOMAS, R., PLANT, M., PLANT, M. and SALES, D. (1989) 'Risks of AIDS among Workers in the "Sex Industry": Some Initial Results from a Scottish Study', *British Medical Journal*, 299, pp. 148–9.

OPPENHEIM, C. (1990) *Poverty: the facts*, London, Child Poverty Action Group.

PATEMAN, C. (1988) *The Sexual Contract*, Cambridge, Polity Press.

PLANT, M. (1990) 'Sex Work, Alcohol, Drugs and AIDS', in M. PLANT (Ed.) *AIDS, Drugs and Prostitution*, London, Routledge.

PLANT, M. (Ed.) (1990) *Aids, Drugs and Prostitution*, London, Routledge.

ROSENBERG, M. and WEINER, J. (1988) 'Prostitutes and AIDS: Health Department Priority?' *American Journal of Public Health*, 78, pp. 418–22.

SCAMBLER, G. (1987) 'Habermas and the Power of Medical Expertise', in G. SCAMBLER (Ed.), *Sociological Theory and Medical Sociology*, London, Tavistock.

SCAMBLER, G., PESWANI, R., RENTON, A. and SCAMBLER, A. (1990) 'Women Prostitutes in the AIDS Era', *Sociology of Health and Illness*, 12, pp. 260–72.
SCOTT, A. (1990) *Ideology and the New Social Movements*, London, Unwin Hyman.
VENEMA, P. and VISSER, J. (1990) 'Safer Prostitution: A New Approach in Holland', in M. PLANT (Ed.), *AIDS, Drugs and Prostitution*, London, Routledge.
WALKOWITZ, J. (1980) *Prostitution and Victorian Society: Women, Class and the State*, New York, Cambridge University Press.
WELLS, J. (1982) *A Herstory of Prostitution in Western Europe*, Berkeley, Calif., Shameless Hussy Press.

6 Sexual Risk among Amphetamine Misusers: Prospects for Change

Hilary Klee

The particular allure of amphetamine sulphate is that it is an antidote to so many unwelcome human conditions. As a stimulant that affects the nervous system rather like adrenaline, it boosts energy levels and alertness, elevates mood, combats obesity and even helps nasal congestion. The medical profession in the UK recognized its value and prescribed it extensively from the 1930s. Those fighting in World War II were often kept going with a supply of 'pep-pills', as they became known. Long-distance lorry drivers, women with weight problems, athletes, students taking examinations — all have used it, and for some time it was the only medication for depression. Despite some unpleasant side effects such as amphetamine psychosis, periodic aggressive outbursts and cardio-vascular disorders that were observed when taken to excess, the demand for amphetamines has remained high. However, the potential for abuse was ultimately acknowledged by the authorities and in 1957 the drug became available only on prescription. There followed an 'epidemic' of illicit use in the 1960s, particularly among some young adults. The situation was much the same in Sweden, Japan, Canada and the United States. Today, amphetamine sulphate's use is ubiquitous across much of the developed world. Much cheaper than cocaine, which tends to be regarded as the 'champagne' of stimulants, it is second only to cannabis in the extent of its use.

It is surprising that a drug with such a history has avoided the attention and disapprobation of British society for so long. Cannabis, heroin and cocaine attract high profile media coverage, which is largely precipitated by drugs seizures associated with very large sums of money. However, drug workers and drugs squads in many parts of the country feel they are witnessing a degree of escalation in amphetamine use that is beyond the control of already overstretched resources. The AIDS epidemic has sharpened awareness that an injectable drug which is highly popular among young people should be a source of grave concern. In the public consciousness, however, concern about a link between HIV transmission and injectable drugs is most often voiced in relation to heroin use.

The first experiences with amphetamine normally involve oral or nasal use (snorting). Some will go on to inject. The injection of amphetamine has advantages over oral use — there is a 'rush' of euphoric, quasi-orgasmic sensation following an injection, and injecting is more economical since little is wasted, an important consideration when you have only a small amount of the drug.[1] The relevance of amphetamine sulphate for HIV transmission is twofold: first, it has a reputation for releasing sexual inhibitions; second, it is a drug that is being injected by large numbers of people. On the one hand there is the risk of sexual transmission, on the other the opportunities to share contaminated injecting equipment.

These considerations, and some preliminary pilot work embedded in a previous study of injecting opiate users (Klee *et al.*, 1990a), led to the research described here. The relatively small group of amphetamine users included in that sample behaved in ways that were different from the larger group of heroin users. For example, the extent of sharing needles and syringes was greater. Motivations were different too. Sharing was not a consequence of desperation for an injection when experiencing withdrawal symptoms; the sharing of amphetamine users tended to relate to group involvement, and the norms associated with it, in a much more pronounced way than was the case with heroin users. They were not only a more sociable group; they were also considerably more sexually active. In this chapter data on the sexual behaviour of amphetamine users are reported, drawn from a study that investigates their lifestyles in more depth.

The Study

The aims of this study were to investigate the sexual and social lifestyles of misusers of amphetamine sulphate in order to assess their potential for contracting and transmitting HIV infection. To this end variables were investigated which included: drug history, current drug use, sexual partnerships, sexual behaviour, the use of condoms, group membership and group activities.

Methods

Data were collected by research assistants using a semi-structured schedule in face-to-face interviews. Interviews lasted between fifty minutes and two hours and were recorded on tape. Responses to questions were subsequently transferred onto coding frames for statistical analysis. Verbatim material was also recorded at this time. The study is ongoing; the data presented here are the results of preliminary analyses of the first phase of the project. More detailed profiles of the behaviour of sub-groups is planned. A second phase of the study, now underway, involves recontacting respondents in order to monitor any changes in drug use and in other variables. Interviews were conducted across the north-west region of England, an area that comprises the cities of Manchester and Liverpool, their suburbs, and towns such as Chester, Bolton and Wigan.

Sample Characteristics

Two hundred amphetamine users were interviewed, 110 injecting, ninety administering the drug orally or nasally. The inclusion of a large proportion of non-injectors allows us to identify the behaviour of the more occasional users and to watch for possible progressions to injecting occurring between first and second interviews. Access to respondents was primarily through streetwork, that is, networking or 'snowballing' using drug users and dealers as mediators for contact with others. Eighty-seven per cent were obtained in this way, another 10 per cent through drug clinics and 3 per cent through the probation services. Ages ranged from 15 to 45 years with 35 per cent under 20, 38 per cent between 20 and 25, and 27 per cent over 25 years. The age profile of this sample is lower than most studies of opiate users partly because opiate research has tended to use clinics as contact points, and partly because amphetamine is used by the young. Seventy per cent of respondents were male and 30 per cent female, a ratio in line with rough estimates of the general population made by drug workers, and consistent with reports from many other drug use studies (Berridge, 1990).

Perceived Effects of Amphetamine Sulphate on Sexual Behaviour

The majority (61 per cent) of respondents reported that using amphetamine increased their interest in sex. A third said the drug had no effect and 6 per cent that their interest decreased. This is in stark contrast to responses to the same question made by opiate users. In previous research, conducted in the same area and using the same methodology, 62 per cent of a sample of 264 opiate users reported *reduced* interest (Klee *et al.*, 1990b).

In the present study respondents over the age of 25 were significantly more likely to say interest increased (74 per cent) than those between 20 and 25 (55 per cent) and the under 20s (52 per cent) (chi-square = 6.94, d.f. = 2, p. −0.03). It may be that the effects on a declining sexual libido are more noticeable, or that the younger respondents were using the drug in contexts where sex was not an option. Weekend use of amphetamine at discos or 'raves' was very popular among younger users whose main aim was to keep dancing as long as possible. From informal observation it seems that amphetamine is taken by the younger, occasional user purely to function with confidence in certain environments, particularly when dancing but also when simply going out 'for a laugh' with 'mates'. Sex is not part of these public environments. The increased interest reported is therefore highly context-dependent.

Injectors were also more likely to report an increase in interest in sex (66 per cent vs 52 per cent for non-injectors, chi-square = 6.57, d.f. = 2, p = 0.045), but this is largely due to a confounding of age with injecting status — predictably a higher proportion of non-injectors were found in the under 20 years age group. It seems that interest is enhanced most for the older users who inject.

The range of effects of amphetamine on sexual performance that were mentioned included both positive and negative aspects, but the positive effects were reported more frequently. Energy was most frequently mentioned as an important benefit by both males (43 per cent) and females (42 per cent), accompanied by anecdotes about sustained sexual activity of olympic proportions. The effects upon sexual orgasm tended to relate to delay in ejaculation. This was seen as positive by 38 per cent of males (and 16 per cent of females who were presumably referring to their amphetamine using partners), but was seen by other males (9 per cent) to be a disadvantage. Some males (36 per cent) had experienced lack of penile erection at a critical moment. As one young man ruefully observed,

Table 1. Gender Differences in the Perceived Effects of Amphetamine on Sexual Performance

| | Effects | | | |
	None	Mixed	Positive	Total
Male	13 (11)	49 (40)	59 (49)	121
Female	8 (16)	4 (8)	38 (76)	50
Total	21 (12)	53 (31)	97 (57)	171

Notes: Row percentages are in parentheses. Data are from respondents who had sexual intercourse while under the influence of amphetamine.

'sometimes you can't get it up and sometimes it's up but it won't go down.' All of these effects have been documented previously on American samples (Grinspoon and Hedblom, 1975; Smith et al., 1979). When respondents were grouped into those who reported wholly positive, those who reported mixed positive and negative, and those who reported no effects (no one reported wholly negative effects), the result was a pronounced gender difference (see Table 1) with females being significantly more likely to be wholly positive about the effects on sexual performance (chi-square = 8.98, d.f. = 2, p = 0.002). However, this observation needs to be interpreted with some caution since most (73 per cent) females in the sample had 'speed'-using regular partners in comparison to 25 per cent of the males. The positive nature of their experiences is likely to have been influenced by the capabilities of their partners. Nevertheless, there are implications here for the sexual risk behaviour of women amphetamine users. We heard several accounts, from both men and women, of women's drinks deliberately being laced with amphetamine, or women being offered amphetamine in order to induce sexual availability, although we have no record of how successful these were.

Amphetamine as a sexual disinhibitor was often referred to, though not always claimed as part of personal experience. The enhanced creativity that was an effect of the drug claimed by some may have extended to sex. Hints of unusual extemporizations were made: 'Speed gets you thinking perverted . . . and very kinky things . . . and you try them out.' Disinhibition seemed to be a property of the drug particularly enjoyed by women. Twenty-five per cent of women reported disinhibition compared to 6 per cent of the men. In general, our impression was that the effects, positive or negative, were often treated with a great deal of humour; reticence was a problem only with some of the very young men.

The Frequency and Recency of Sexual Intercourse

The frequency and recency of sexual intercourse are shown in Table 2. Without comparative data from non-drug users of similar ages, it is impossible to say whether these figures suggest a higher than average level of sexual activity. It is clear, however, that sexual intercourse for this group is considerably greater than for comparative groups of opiate users.

Comparing respondents injecting amphetamine in the current study with opiate injectors in the Klee et al. (1990b) study, only 54 per cent of opiate injectors

Table 2   The Recency and Frequency of Sexual Intercourse in the Six Months Prior to Interview

Recency		Frequency*	
< 1 month	152 (80%)	4–7 times p/w	52 (27%)
< 6 months	23 (12%)	2–3 times p/w	63 (33%)
> 6 months	15 (8%)	once p/w or less	64 (34%)
		none	11 (6%)

Notes: * Average over the period. Missing values = 10.

Table 3   The Relationship between Injecting Status, Sharing and Casual Sexual Encounters in the Six Months Prior to Interview

	Injecting		Sharing* Yes No		Not injecting
Casual sex	Yes	58 (53)	29	29	36 (40)
	No	52 (47)	31	20	53 (60)
Total		110	60	49	89

Notes: Column percentages are in parentheses.
* Missing values = 1.

had engaged in sexual intercourse within the previous month compared to 80 per cent of amphetamine injectors. The contrast is even more marked for the frequency of intercourse. Thirty-nine per cent of the opiate injectors reported no sexual activity in the previous six months, compared to 6 per cent of amphetamine injectors. A frequency of once per week or more was reported by 33 per cent of opiate injectors, and a rate of twice a week or more by 60 per cent of amphetamine injectors. These figures suggest that the potential for the sexual transmission of HIV by amphetamine users is considerably greater than that of opiate users.

Casual Sex

Frequent casual sexual encounters may be a source of risk if condoms are not used. Table 3 shows the proportions of injecting and non-injecting respondents who reported such encounters in the six months prior to interview. The table also shows the numbers who had used others' injecting equipment in the same period. Half of those injecting respondents who reported casual sex (*N* = 58) had shared their needles and syringes.

Sex without Condoms

Unless condoms are used, there is potential for the transmission of infection. The number of occasions of unprotected sexual intercourse in the six months prior to interview for the respondents who were sexually active in that period is shown in Table 4. The sexual activity of the respondents not reporting casual sex refers

Table 4   The Relationship between the Number of Occasions of Unprotected Sexual Intercourse and Casual Sex in the Six Months Prior to Interview

| | Intercourse without condoms | | | | |
	None*	< 20	< 50	> 50	Total
Casual sex					
Yes	5 (6)	37 (45)	17 (20)	24 (29)	83
No	9 (11)	13 (16)	23 (27)	39 (46)	84
Total	14 (8)	50 (30)	40 (24)	63 (38)	167

Notes: Row percentages are in parentheses. Missing values = 8. *Condoms used every time

exclusively to intercourse with a regular partner. A total of fourteen respondents (8 per cent of all sexually active respondents for whom we have data) said they did not have unprotected sexual intercourse and that they used condoms every time. Only five (6 per cent) of those reporting casual sex used condoms every time. Ninety-four per cent of this group reported a number of unprotected sexual episodes. However, the table also shows, perhaps predictably, that those whose sexual activity was only with regular partners reported the highest incidence of sex without condoms (46 per cent vs 29 per cent, chi-square = 17.13, d.f. = 3, p = 0.001).

Attitudes to Condoms

Thirty-seven per cent of respondents had never used condoms, 24 per cent had used them but not for over a year, 29 per cent had used them in the last year. Sixty-four percent disliked them, 26 per cent were neutral and 10 per cent were fairly happy about using them. These data include the views of those who volunteered an opinion about the acceptability of condoms despite the fact that they had never used them.

It was interesting to find that there were no significant gender differences in condom acceptability since in the Klee et al. (1990b) study female opiate users disliked them less than did men. It may be that the relatively negative response of 'speed' using women to condoms is related to their more active sexual role.

Ten per cent of respondents had experienced problems of awkwardness or embarrassment when using condoms, for 18 per cent problems were of a more mechanical nature (bursting, slipping off), while 72 per cent reported that they had experienced no problems at all. No significant statistical relationship was found between negative experiences and the degree of acceptability.

Amphetamine and Alcohol

Forty-three per cent of the sample described themselves as regular users of alcohol; of these a quarter used amphetamine to delay inebriation and to be able to drink more. A significant relationship was found between casual sex and the use of 'speed' to increase alcohol tolerance. Eighty-two per cent of this group reported casual sexual encounters in the six months prior to interview in comparison with

54 per cent of the respondents not using the drug in this way (chi-square = 5.20, d.f. = 1, p = 0.023). They tend to be young unattached men who like to go to clubs or pubs with their friends. The greater incidence of casual sex may be accounted for partly by their availability as prospective partners, but the combination of these substances may be an enhancing factor.

Prospects for Behavioural Change

Despite the preliminary nature of these analyses, the results suggest that amphetamine users should be more prominent targets for health promotion strategies. They are sexually highly active, mostly young, and many are injecting the drug. Over half of the injectors in this sample had used others' injecting equipment in the previous six months. Amphetamine has the potential for enhancing sexual disinhibition, and this combines with the typically social function that the drug performs to produce a psychological and social environment conducive to sexual risk.

There is a variety of impediments in the way of decreasing the use of amphetamine, and of eliminating the sharing of injecting equipment. A decline in amphetamine misuse seems unlikely in the near future. The drug is cheaper, more easily available and less detectable in behavioural terms than many other illicit drugs. For most users it is highly functional, and its power to elevate mood and increase energy is highly valued. It does not have the social stigma attached to other drugs like heroin nor the reputation for addictive properties. Its facilitation of social interaction may be a factor that contributes to the sharing of injecting equipment, though analysis of these issues has yet to be performed on these data.

The picture is similarly unpromising with regard to the use of condoms. Despite consistent attempts to convert the sexually 'at risk' population to them since the AIDS epidemic started, there is little evidence of comprehensive and sustained use of condoms. This is as true of amphetamine misusers as it is of other groups in society. The connection between HIV infection and condoms may backfire — proposing to use one implies HIV risk, and foregrounds something that neither party wishes to contemplate. It was noticeable in both this research and the previous study of opiate users that the risk of HIV was associated more with injecting drugs than with having sex.

The prospects of behavioural change are rather bleak, but certain courses of action could be tried. Amphetamine users are unlikely to venture into drug units, clinics and even drop-in centres, despite strenuous attempts by many drug workers to make them user-friendly since they rarely offer appropriate treatment. Such places are associated with 'smack-heads' (heroin users). The opportunities for the communication of harm reduction messages are thus limited. However, outreach workers have succeeded in making contact in some areas. Resources are needed to allow for further efforts in this direction. Additionally, the exclusive link between heroin and HIV risk in the minds of young drug users needs to be broken and the dangers of injecting amphetamine addressed more directly in future campaigns.

Finally, it has become apparent in this research that large networks of amphetamine users exist. Linked groups within regions often have several members who are identifiable leaders. Some are small-time dealers with a large clientele. Others are simply gregarious people who enjoy having people to visit and keep 'open house'. The characteristics of these key figures vary but they are similar in the considerable influence they exert over the lives of the others in the group. Unfortunately, there is too little research in this area to offer anything more than a suggestion about their potential as facilitators or effectors of behavioural change. If group norms are to change with respect to injecting and sexual risk, it seems likely that the changes will start here. They have a role as opinion leaders, and if they can be convinced of the desirability of certain health preserving acts, they may be more successful in initiating behavioural change than any experienced drug worker.

At present amphetamine users seem beyond the reach of health professionals. Much stands in the way of such contact, but perhaps the task of health educators will be made easier if key targets are defined and outreach work is aimed directly at them.

Acknowledgments

The project is funded by the Economic and Social Research Council. The data were collected by Cath Hayes, Barbara Nodwell and Alex Howie.

Note

1 There may be another advantage too for some, though this is more speculative; this is the effect on self-esteem of acquiring a paramedical skill. For the young unemployed with few ways to demonstrate personal competence, this, and the ritual associated with assembling and using injecting paraphernalia, may add to the attraction.

References

BERRIDGE, V. (1990) (Ed.) *Drugs Research and Policy in Britain*, London, Avebury.
GRINSPOON, L. and HEDBLOM, P. (1975) *The Speed Culture: Amphetamine Use and Abuse in America*, Cambridge Mass., Harvard University Press.
KLEE, H., FAUGIER, J. and MORRIS, J. (1990a) Intravenous drug users: their role in the sexual mediation of HIV infection. Final report to the Economic and Social Research Council.
KLEE, H., FAUGIER, J., MORRIS, J., HAYES, C. and BOULTON, T. (1990b) Sexual partners of injecting drug users: the risk of HIV infection. *British Journal of Addiction*, 85, pp. 413–418.
SMITH, D.E., BUXTON, M.E. and DAMMAN, G. (1979) Amphetamine abuse and sexual dysfunction. In D.E. SMITH (Ed.) *Amphetamine Use, Misuse and Abuse*, Boston, Mass., G.K. Hall & Co.

7   HIV/AIDS Knowledge and Migrant Workers*

Mary Haour-Knipe, Sofi Ospina, François Fleury and Erwin Zimmermann

Switzerland has always been linked in one way or another with the phenomenon of migration. Today, with the exception of Luxembourg, Switzerland is the European country with the highest proportion of foreign inhabitants, some 16 per cent of the resident population. Swiss policy does not particularly favour the acquisition of citizenship, thus many of these are second or third generation immigrants to live in the country. Although 180 different countries are represented, all but 12 per cent of foreign residents are from other European countries, about two-fifths being Italians who arrived in a wave of labour migration in the 1960s and 1970s.

The country also hosts migrants of other kinds, including employees of international organizations, and, as in all other European countries, an increasing number of persons seeking asylum as well as an unknown, but significant, number of clandestine migrants. A further category of migrant worker is the 'seasonal worker', who spends nine months working in the country and returns home annually for the remaining three months. Seasonal workers are not allowed to bring family members with them; they provide a relatively inexpensive and easily administered source of labour since annual quotas can be fixed according to economic conditions.

HIV/AIDS Evaluation

Switzerland is one of the few countries in the world to have well evaluated HIV/AIDS education campaigns. A first wave of studies, starting with a before and after telephone survey of the effects of a brochure distributed to all households in 1986, has been following by annual studies among gay and bisexual men and injecting drug users, and also among young people, heterosexual adults, sex tourists, dropouts and hospital workers.

* This study was funded by the Swiss Federal Public Health Office, Study, 1.6, 'Les migrants: Saisonniers portugais et espagnols'.

These studies had shown that the general populations and specific groups were reasonably well informed, and had increasingly adopted protective behaviours (Dubois-Arber *et al.*, 1989; Stutz and Zimmermann, 1990). It was not at all certain, however, whether a similar situation pertained among foreign residents. An early study of AIDS-related knowledge and behaviours among this migrant population thus took place in 1988 among Turkish asylum seekers and African students (Fleury *et al.*, 1991). The Turkish segment of this study continues. The focus of this chapter is on a second study which has looked at seasonal workers. The emphasis is on this group because it was assumed that more settled foreign populations had probably been reached by 'general population' HIV/AIDS education campaigns. Clandestine populations, although possibly poorly informed, are very difficult to reach. We therefore decided to focus attention on a task at which we thought we had a reasonable chance of success.

The situation of the seasonal worker is fairly well known in Switzerland (Steinauer, 1980). Many of those who originally came as seasonal workers in the 1960s have long since earned the legal right to bring their families and are assimilated into Swiss society. More recent seasonal workers alternate three months in the home country with nine months of work in Switzerland, in a cycle often repeated for many years. They thus live to some extent on the margins of two or more cultures, absent from home for most of the year and poorly, or not at all, integrated in Switzerland.

About half work in the construction industry, with a further 30 per cent in the hotel industry (most of the women hired as seasonal workers are employed in this sector). In theory an individual is given a contract for a specific job, but in practice there is a certain amount of movement among jobs, employment sector and legal status. It is not uncommon, for example, for someone to work in a hotel for a few months during the ski season, stay on as a 'tourist', then work for a few months during the summer on a construction site. Among the seasonal workers themselves, legal status and previous employment experience in Switzerland determine informal status and power.

Those who work in the construction industry live in barracks with other seasonal workers or in small apartments rented by the employer, while those who work in hotels are usually lodged there. Living with others of the same status, the seasonal worker often has little opportunity to learn, or to speak, the local language. Social life is thus usually among compatriots. There is rarely much contact with Swiss people. In this study we chose to focus on two of the principal national groups of seasonal workers, those from Portugal and those from Spain. Seasonal workers of these nationalities predominate in the French-speaking regions of the country where the research was carried out.

The specific hypotheses under investigation were: (i) seasonal workers would have little knowledge of AIDS, their marginal position in both the country of origin and the host country would mean that they had not been reached to any significant extent by HIV/AIDS information campaigns; (ii) seasonal workers' ambivalent situation in the host culture would lead to a higher incidence of risk behaviours. Specifically, legal restrictions on family reunification (two-thirds are married) would necessitate either sexual abstinence or transitory sexual relationships. Seasonal workers might additionally be more likely clients for the peripheral 'market' of sex workers who may be injecting drug users, and in less of a position to require the use of condoms; and (iii) there would be differences in sexual behaviour according to work site. The holiday atmosphere prevailing in a ski resort may foster transitory sexual relationships between various populations, including the seasonal hotel workers, more so than for construction workers in cities.

Sampling

Conventional probability sampling techniques are unfeasible with mixed migrant populations in which groups shift rapidly and some are in the country clandestinely. Non-probability sampling, in this case snowball sampling using several points of departure, can however create samples which approach representativeness (Martin and Dean, 1990).

A long phase of preparation was necessary before sampling could take place. The first step was to get an overview by reading the available sociological and other literature and talking with appropriate professionals. The second was to contact those involved with seasonal workers, for example trade unions, immigrant associations, directors of barracks and religious leaders. The third stage involved working through key informants in hotels, bars, construction sites, and through personal contacts. Only then were we ready to interview people.

This was done by going to a previously defined site, seasonal workers' living quarters at the end of the dinner hour, for example. For interviews in the ski station, which was a three-hour journey from our home base, a team of four interviewers stayed on site for a week. Having already gained considerable experience recruiting and interviewing, they were able to start the process at the third stage described above, that of defining, then working through key informants.

The best means of accessing interviewees was through personal contact, community leaders and through the barracks. Although officials, even when agreeing to the importance of the problem, had predicted that it would be difficult for seasonal workers to talk about matters related to sexuality and HIV/AIDS, when interviewers reached them and explained the project, seasonal workers inevitably volunteered to participate, and/or recruit a friend who would be willing to do so. Only once did someone categorically refuse, although the occasional person approached said they were 'not interested'. Those who did participate gave a series of reasons: the status or simple good will coming from cooperating with a research project, doing something to help with HIV/AIDS, or less altruistically, simply to talk to somebody, to earn some money, or for something to do in the evening.

Participants were paid a modest sum for participating, and given a 'Stop AIDS' pen to keep, stamped with an address and telephone number from which further information could be obtained. Approximately one in ten respondents refused payment, and some spontaneously offered to contribute money towards a prevention campaign oriented towards seasonal workers.

The various approaches described above, with at least twenty sample recruitment points, offer a diversity of sites and personalities which should make any biases cancel one another. Only one source of possible bias would seem to be systematic: given the manner of recruiting research subjects by asking for volunteers from among a group, the sample may be biased in the direction of people already interested in HIV/AIDS. It would have been easy for someone with negative feelings about the syndrome, for example, to have avoided being approached.

Data Collection Techniques

Two data collection techniques were used simultaneously, semi-structured interviews and standardized questionnaires. The semi-structured interview (fifty-eight subjects) lasted about one hour and covered impressions retained from HIV/AIDS education campaigns in the home and host countries; knowledge and attitudes related to HIV, AIDS, STDs, and condoms; family, sex education, social and sexual life in the home and host countries; and attitudes and ideas concerning marriage, virginity, fidelity, injecting drug use, same gender sexual activity and commercial sex workers. All but seven of those interviewed also filled out the standardized questionnaire (the missing questionnaires are attributable to an initial misunderstanding by an interviewer). We can thus compare answers obtained by two different methods from fifty-one subjects. An additional 111 people filled out the questionnaire only.

The questionnaire (158 subjects) was a standard KABP-type model developed from various sources (WHO, 1988; IPSO, 1989), adapted and translated from English and French into Spanish, tested, revised, back-translated into French to test the appropriateness of the language, re-tested and revised. The Portuguese version was translated from the Spanish version, and also back-translated and tested before reaching its final form. This long and complicated process was necessary to make sure the translations were culturally appropriate and understood.

The role of the interviewers was critical when approaching seasonal workers. It was necessary to find Spanish- and Portuguese-speaking people who would be capable of interviewing, among others, construction workers about, among other things, their sexual lives; and of handling whatever might come up in the interview. It was felt important that the interviewers not only speak the same language as the interviewees, but also be in a recognizably similar situation. One member of the research team is a Spanish-speaking Latin American. Three of the other four interviewers were also Latin American graduate students and academics, and one of the first Portuguese interviewees later did interviews with three of his compatriots. For the Spanish respondents, particularly, it turned out to be helpful that the interviewers were apart from regional rivalries and stereotypes.

We had been concerned, for several reasons, about the sex of the interviewer. Would it be possible for women interviewers to gather information from men about their sexuality without getting themselves into ambiguous situations, especially if the interview took place in bars or in man's living quarters? Could a male interviewer do good interviews with women subjects? The second question is rapidly answered with a 'yes': about half of the interviews with the Spanish women were done by a man, with no noticeable difference in the quality of the information gathered. The answer to the first question is also 'yes', but not without due precaution. Female interviewers were talking about sex to men who may live their daily lives with other men and who have little everyday contact with women, and certainly have little familiarity with women researchers. If none of the three women interviewers had any difficulty, this was largely because they themselves were very clear about their roles as researchers, and about projecting this role and no other. The were careful about how they dressed for an interview, for example, and were firm in rejecting advances on the few occasions an interviewee failed to understand.

It was felt ethically wrong to collect information without doing HIV/AIDS prevention work in return. After each interview, the interviewer therefore stayed to discuss and answer questions if there were any. Members of the research team also met individually and as a group with all of the interviewers several times, discussing the research, but mainly teaching about HIV and about AIDS, so they could answer questions which might arise during or after the interviews. We also tracked each of the interviewers quite carefully in the beginning, making sure he or she had one of the research team available by telephone if necessary, 'debriefing' by listening to an interviewer's first tapes and discussing them afterwards.

Findings

The population studied consists of twenty-nine Spanish and twenty-nine Portuguese interviewed, and of seventy-nine individuals of each nationality who answered the questionnaire. Men comprise 78 per cent of the sample, which makes it representative for Portuguese seasonal workers (81 per cent male). Spanish women are slightly overrepresented (22 per cent, versus 10 per cent in the overall population of seasonal workers). The mean age for the Spanish is 29 years, and 27 for the Portuguese. A third of the sample is married, in contrast with two-thirds of the general Hispano-Portuguese seasonal worker population in Switzerland.

For about half of the sample, schooling did not go beyond the primary level: some had been to school for only two or three years, whereas one or two had some university education. Most of those studied had been coming to work in Switzerland for several years.

The sample is representative with regard to the socio-demographic characteristics of the population of Spanish and Portuguese seasonal workers in Switzerland, with the following exceptions: our population is a little younger and less often married. Women, especially Spanish women, are overrepresented. Those working in the hotel industry in the ski resort are also oversampled, in accordance with the hypothesis concerning behaviour differences according to work site.

What do seasonal workers know about 'AIDS'? Does the fact that they migrate without their families for temporary stays affect their risk? And what results are brought by quantitative versus qualitative methodologies? In this chapter, rather than comparing the sample to another population, we compare it to itself, using two different methodologies. Nationality, sex and other pertinent differences between the groups studied are mentioned in the text when applicable.

Quantitative Data

Having recruited the sample by asking people to participate in a study about AIDS, it comes as no surprise that we found nobody who was not aware of the syndrome. In response to the questionnaire, almost 60 per cent said they were somewhat to very concerned about the problem, and eight Spanish and five Portuguese reported knowing one or more people affected.

All in all, seasonal workers' 'AIDS knowledge' was relatively good. The principal modes of transmission, unprotected sex and exchanging syringes, are known by over 90 per cent of those having filled out questionnaires. There is some lingering doubt over blood transfusions, specifically restricted in the

Table 1   Seasonal Workers' AIDS Knowledge: Modes of HIV Transmission

'AIDS can be transmitted by':	yes (percentages)
sex act	95
re-using syringes	90
blood transfusion	71
at the dentist	40
at the hairdresser	25
insect bites	36
deep kissing	17
shaking hands	4
in public transportation	7
using public toilets	33
public swimming pools	22
re-using a drinking glass	27
coughing	13
'Protection by'	**yes (percentages)**
use condoms	94
sexual fidelity	75
don't inject	76
don't re-use syringe	73
vaccination	48
blood test	71

questionnaire to a blood transfusion in Switzerland, where routine testing of the blood supply has been in effect since 1985, but less than half of the respondents think 'AIDS' can be transmitted at the dentist, and only a quarter at the hairdresser. About a third think HIV can be transmitted by insect bites.

Responses to the 'public toilets' item in the questionnaire were hard to interpret since, as a respondent had pointed out in the pilot phase of the study, public toilets used for unprotected sex may indeed be places of possible transmission. Even putting this on one side, zones of ambiguity remain in the 'ordinary acts of everyday life' category. For some, 'AIDS' is thought to be 'caught' swimming in public pools or by re-using drinking glasses.

As for protection, almost all respondents cited condoms. Condoms have been heavily promoted in the pragmatic Swiss prevention campaigns, less so in the countries of origin of our research subject, where there have been difficulties with this specific prevention message. We also find relatively good results for 'sexual fidelity' as a means of prevention, another key component in Swiss campaigns for an interval, as well as for the drug-related items: not injecting and not re-using syringes. On the other hand, almost half of the respondents think they can be protected against HIV with a vaccination which does not yet exist. As for sexual partnership behaviour, on the questionnaire respondents reported sexual relations within the past six months as shown in Table 2.

The data have to be interpreted with considerable caution since several extraneous factors may have affected the responses. For example, seasonal workers arrive in the host country at different intervals during the year depending on where they are to work, and whether the questionnaire was administered a few

Table 2 *Sexual Partners and Condom Use in the Past Six Months*

	None		Stable partners		Transitory relations		Total
Total	35	(23)	69	(45)	49	(32)	100%
Men	22	(19)	55	(46)	42	(35)	100%
Women	13	(38)	14	(41)	7	(21)	100%
Condom use							
never	6	(67)	38	(61)	16	(32)	N = 60
sometimes	2	(22)	15	(24)	23	(46)	N = 40
always	1	(11)	9	(15)	11	(22)	N = 21
Total	9	(100)	62	(100)	50	(100)	

Note: Percentages are shown in brackets.

weeks or a few months after arrival may make a difference to responses concerning sexual behaviour.

Of interest for the purposes of studying potential HIV risk is the transitory relations column. In this category are forty-nine individuals who responded that in the past six months they had sexual relationship(s) with other than, or in addition to, a spouse or a 'stable partner'. Proportionally more men than women put themselves in this category. Half are between 20 and 29 years of age, and they are less likely than their counterparts to be married. Nine men indicate on the questionnaire that they have used the services of a sex worker. As for ski resort behaviour compared with that in other sites, nine out of twenty-eight (32 per cent) questionnaires filled out in the ski resort place the respondent in the transitory relations category, compared with thirty-nine out of 127 (31 per cent) in the other locations, a non-significant difference. Finally, for protection behaviours, half of the sample never uses condoms. More pertinently, about a third of those having transitory sexual relationships do so without condoms, and an additional half use them only 'sometimes' on such occasions. Condoms are always used during transitory sexual relationships by less than a quarter of the sample.

Qualitative Data

Our qualitative data come from fifty-eight semi-directive interviews and from ethnographic observations of the ski resort by a team of four interviewers. The first point to be reported in the previous section was that many interviewees were quite concerned about 'AIDS'. Interview data elaborates: if the main source of information for most was the media, particularly television and newspapers, there is clear indication that an individual's degree of concern is largely a matter of propinquity. The more someone had been personally touched by the phenomenon of AIDS, the greater his or her concern.

Thus personalized 'stories' were talked about vividly, no matter what the source. Especially remembered were television programmes, as was the Spanish 'Diary of a Seropositive' still mentioned two years after its distribution. For many respondents however, the point at which they became aware of the disease was at

Table 3 Spontaneously Mentioned Modes of HIV Transmission and Protection

Transmission	(N = 58)	Protection	
Sex in general	43	Condom	28
Injection of drugs	26	Careful partner choice and/or hygiene	11
Contact with blood	17	Blood test	11
Blood transfusion	14	Fidelity	11
Homosexual relations	10		

the death of American movie actor Rock Hudson. A few interviewees had been directly affected by the syndrome. One 22-year-old musician, for example, was working for the second season as an agricultural worker in Switzerland. Both his motivations and his plans were complex, but more or less explicitly included an attempt to break away from the drug scene in a large urban area in his home country. He reported knowing four people affected by AIDS, his HIV/AIDS knowledge was correct and detailed, and he reported that his behaviour has changed in that he now always uses condoms.

Specific knowledge concerning HIV transmission and protection was gathered in response to open questions, thus reflecting what the research subjects thought, as compared to what the researchers thought they might think when the questionnaire was designed. Table 3 shows, in decreasing order of importance, spontaneously respondents thought 'AIDS' could be transmitted and how people mentioned ways in which could protect themselves.

Modes of transmission mentioned spontaneously in response to an open question are thus similar to those assessed by the standardized questionnaire, with the addition of a 'contact with blood' item concerning somehow touching or being contaminated with blood. Three people (two women) also spontaneously mentioned mother to child transmission. Several interviewees correctly pointed out that the host country has one of the highest incidences of AIDS in Europe, and that they therefore have to be particularly careful.

In relation to protection, almost half the interviewees spontaneously mentioned condoms, but eleven people (19 per cent), without notable difference by nationality or by sex, felt that a good way to protect themselves against 'AIDS' is to be careful in the choice of sexual partner, and/or to pay special attention to hygiene.

The interview data contain a wealth of images about HIV and AIDS. Within our sample of migrant workers we find the entire range of comprehension, from excellent (one Portuguese man stated that AIDS is an immunodeficiency syndrome) to appalling (another respondent stated that he knows someone with AIDS and is afraid she will fall down dead in front of him). Drawing a parallel between AIDS and cancer, an analogy made by several interviewees, a Spanish interviewee said that AIDS is caused by a virus, a disease that 'eats one up from inside'.

Traces of scientific debates just prior to the winter of 1989–90 when the interviews took place are present. For example, one person, a hairdresser, pointed out that his work put him at risk, another mentioned razor blades, and two mentioned ear piercing. Two interviewees, both women, spoke of having read or heard of medicines: without mentioning compound Q, one woman spoke of a medicine based on plants which might be of help, and another of 'pills which do not cure but which "slow down" the disease but are very expensive. . . .' Finally, five men spoke of a healthy lifestyle as a mode of protection: avoiding alcohol and tobacco, doing sports, and avoiding the abuse of tranquillizers and hypnotics which increase vulnerability. Confidential use of the HIV antibody test as a guide in managing one's own preventive behaviours is promoted in Switzerland, and some interviewees spoke of wishing to know they were HIV seronegative at the beginning of a new relationship. Others spoke of using the test more from the point of view of control, recommending, for example, that all sex workers be tested, or even that everyone be tested every two months.

A contagious disease model was adhered to by a minority of respondents. One person stated that 'AIDS' could be 'caught' from someone else's breath, and another that it could be caught from the wind. One woman thought she might be at risk through picking things up from the ground. At least one person said 'AIDS' could be caught by sitting on a seat left warm by somebody on a bus, another by using a dirty glass or plate, or in the public baths. The interviews, in addition, point to potential confusion between AIDS and other sexually transmitted diseases. A 39-year-old Portuguese man, for example, married with a family in Portugal and a long history of travels around the world, assured the interviewer that AIDS used to be called the clap (a case of which he once picked up 'from a prostitute in Venezuela') and comes from promiscuity and lack of hygiene. He also felt that one may be more or less vulnerable depending on whether one has strong or weak blood.

The task was to evaluate the effectiveness of prevention efforts, not to study illness metaphors and models. Nevertheless, we were struck by how, on the whole, respondents' knowledge reflects the medical science not of a generation ago as popular medical knowledge did twenty or thirty years ago, (c.f. Boltanksi, 1975) but of at most a couple of years ago. Reflecting what was in the scientific press only five years ago, for example, several interviewees said they had heard AIDS started in Africa, and one or two brought up the familiar attribution to green monkeys (see Chapter 3, this volume).

Overall, the interview data were superior to data gathered by questionnaires in helping us understand where further interventions are needed. For example, reassurance is necessary for those who think HIV can be transmitted by ordinary contacts since in this study at least they are the most worried. Certain misconceptions need to be dealt with, for example the belief that good personal hygiene and careful attention to body odours of a prospective sexual partner can protect against HIV transmission. Finally, efforts are needed to reinforce the message that HIV transmission is a matter of risky behaviour rather than of risk group. Several interviewees made reference to sex workers as vectors, as well as people who have numerous sexual partners. One man remarked that a way to protect himself is to go with a woman who is more expensive, another talked of staying at home. One Spanish woman said she had heard that people from Yugoslavia are singled out for HIV testing during the obligatory medical for entry to Switzerland, thereby denigrating the very group replacing the Spanish as seasonal workers in Switzerland at the time the interviews were carried out. One Spanish woman, who has been observing the behaviour of tourists from her vantage point as a hotel worker in a Swiss ski resort for the past eleven years, thought that the English must be particularly at risk.

Behaviour

Semi-structured interviews explored respondents' possible drug use and sexual behaviours. Interviewers did not ask directly about drug use, but introduced the subject in general terms, and let the respondent react as he or she wished, probing as appropriate. One or two people hinted at having injected drugs in the past (one example is cited earlier), and several others mentioned the occasional use of marijuana and hashish. There is no indication, though, that any of those interviewed were currently injecting drugs, even occasionally.

Concerning sexual behaviour, interview questions were also indirect: neither in setting up the interview guide nor once fieldwork had begun did interviewers feel comfortable asking direct questions, because the cultures of the populations studied do not permit easy discussion of sexual matters with strangers, and because, for the same reasons, we doubted the reliability and validity of information forthcoming. The occasional respondent spoke directly about his or her own behaviour without being asked, but this was relatively rare. Coding the interview data concerning sexual behaviour required a certain amount of reading between the lines, but in most cases a given individual's 'story' was coherent enough for three members of the research team to agree on a category.

Interview data and questionnaire data concerning sexual behaviour tell quite different stories. Without extrapolating beyond the data, it seems clear that in the interviews respondents of both sexes bias replies in the direction they think is socially desirable or expected. Thus, in this Latin European sample, a little over half of the women leave an impression of sexual abstinence, while a similar proportion of men claim to have had transitory sexual relations. Both of these proportions decrease in the questionnaire. It is interesting to note that the proportion of those who commit themselves to avowing what is less socially acceptable for their sex remains the same with both methodologies: 23 per cent of women report transitory relationships in the interview and 21 per cent on the questionnaire, whereas 17 per cent of the men report abstinence in the interviews and 18 per cent in the questionnaire.

A perhaps prototypic example is a man for whom we have data collected using three different methods. In a group interview during the pilot phase of the study he talked a great deal about his numerous sexual 'conquests', as well as the large number of sex workers he had visited. On the questionnaire, filled out after the group interview, in contrast, he said he had not had sexual relations in the past six months. In interview, he turned out to be a young man on a lengthy sick leave from his job as a construction worker, and wanting only to return home. His reasons for staying in his room in the evenings, he said, were that the sickness insurance people were liable to check on him and also that he had heard that sex workers require condoms, which he does not like, so why bother going out. . . .

All in all, for sexual behaviour, and among the population studied here, the research team felt more confident of the validity of questionnaire than interview data. Research subjects seemed more willing to commit themselves to an anonymous questionnaire than to a face-to-face interviewer. When the two data sources were compared, a given respondent's answers on the questionnaire made more coherent sense with the rest of his or her story.

Interview data did, however, shed light on two major points related to the original hypotheses concerning sex work and ski resort behaviour. It will be

Figure 1   Sexual Behaviour By Sex Interview Data and Questionnaire Data

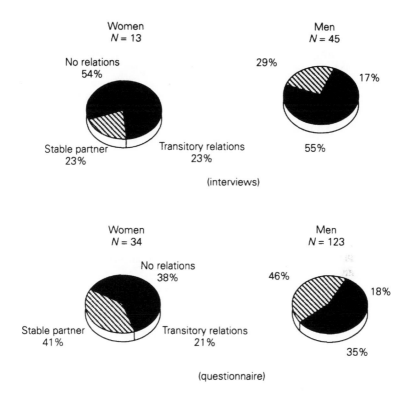

recalled that one of the hypotheses concerned the possibility that seasonal workers would be particularly vulnerable to turning towards the 'grey market' of sex workers possibly involved in injecting drug use. Since this has potentially great significance for HIV transmission, interviewers were instructed to probe in some detail. They began by broaching the subject of sex work in a general manner, gradually becoming more specific by asking if the respondent's friends ever had sex with sex workers, about the price of a visit, about sex work in and around the barracks and about condom use. Although one young man broke off the interview at this point, rare were the others who, after going through all this, did not talk about their own behaviour. Eight interviewees (out of fifty-eight) talked of having visited commercial sex workers, whereas only nine (out of 158) checked having done so on the questionnaire. The former had no time frame imposed whereas the latter was to have specifically concerned only the past six months, but this difference in proportion leads us to believe that projective-type questions were effective in eliciting information about what, among the men studied, was socially a not very unacceptable form of behaviour.

Visiting sex workers was described by the interviewees as being a 'rite de passage' for many young men at some point during their adolescence. Nobody described this as the ideal form of interpersonal relationship; it was usually described as somewhat 'sad' and/or machine-like, requiring a certain dose of alcohol to carry through, and several younger men implied that it would be beneath them to pay for sex. Several of the older married men, on the other hand, visited professional sex workers for physical relief without emotional involvement, in a form of fidelity to their wives in the home country. As for the sensitive issue of 'grey market' sex workers, everybody had heard of them, but nobody had visited one. It became clear in the interviews that visiting a sex worker is a somewhat shameful activity for many seasonal migrant workers, in which he, a guest in the country, feels in a not very powerful demander's position. In this position it is far easier to go to a known area where the situation is unambiguous, and where no negotiation is necessary. An additional factor is that most seasonal workers have only rudimentary mastery of the language of the host country: several said one of the chief advantages of relations with a commercial sex worker is that there is no necessity to speak. Many tourists and foreigners in countries patronize supermarkets rather than markets and small shops for exactly the same reasons.

A final point before turning to protective behaviour concerns rumour and gossip, a possible important source of bias in the study in general, as also an important element for understanding behaviour in the ski resort. Just as interviewees tended to bias what they told the interviewer about their behaviour in the direction of socially acceptable behaviour, there was a tendency to credit rumour for fact as far as the behaviour of others was concerned, and almost always in the direction of sexual excess rather than the contrary. Gossip tended to inflate everybody else's sexual behaviour, both men's and women's. In analyzing the data, we therefore ignored most of what people said about others' behaviour, and stuck to what the respondent about his or her own comportment.

Neither the interview data, when restricted to what respondents said and implied about their own behaviour, nor the questionnaire data confirmed the hypothesis that a vacation atmosphere and an easier mixing of populations (both sexes work and live together in the hotel) lead to more frequent casual sexual relations among migrant workers in the ski resort. Interviewees explained that there are several reasons for this. First, resort patrons were described as 'racist': there is little mingling between clients and staff. Second, hotel and restaurant work is hard, hours are long and irregular, and if clients are on holiday, staff most definitely are not. In addition, it is quite possible that free time falls when all one's acquaintances are working. As with hospital personnel and others with irregular hours, social life thus tends to be restricted to colleagues.

It is here that social control was described as being very strong indeed. The ski resort, from the point of view of the 100 or so seasonal workers employed there, was described as a village. Everybody knows everybody else, and it is difficult to escape from the observation of compatriots, especially since people congregate in the same places in the evening. In a word, among the populations studied here, the women, especially, are strongly discouraged from engaging in transitory sexual relationships so as not to be talked about.

Attitudes

Overall, the majority of both Spanish and Portuguese respondents who expressed an opinion spoke of the need for solidarity with people affected by AIDS, making statements such as 'we should not turn our backs', or 'we should help people', or finally, 'it must be terrible to know you are going to die'. Only four people said they would drop a friend they discovered had HIV/AIDS. The vast majority said they would work with someone who had HIV/AIDS, and only one out of five would refuse to live with somebody affected: the latter, not surprisingly, tended to believe the syndrome can be transmitted by ordinary contact.

The majority of those interviewed expressed liberal attitudes in several domains. With only four exceptions, construction workers and hotel employees were accepting of sex between men. As one respondent put it, 'I have nothing against: everybody should do as they like. I respect their choice. Everybody should be able to define themselves sexually.'

Towards sex workers, attitudes were somewhat less tolerant. About half who expressed an opinion talked of vice and lack of hygiene. The other half, five women and six men, talked of the psychological, familial or financial problems that women who sell sex must have had to make them go into the profession, and of the health and other problems that result.

As for injecting drug users, the interviewees were far more severe. Only one person took an attitude of tolerance and of freedom of choice. Six others argued along psycho-medical lines not untouched by moralism. As two respondents stated, 'Addicts are unhappy people who don't have the strength to get out of it. They let everything go.' 'They are killing themselves. They make me very sad.'

Another respondent talked of the need to keep away from drug users, who represent a danger for the people around them: 'If a friend became an addict I'd leave him. When someone becomes an addict he's lost.' Several people told us of severe drug problems in their villages and cities of origin, and many of those with the least tolerant attitudes had been directly affected.

Towards a Typology of Responses

One advantage of qualitative data is that they allow the elaboration of theories which can be of use in understanding the link between knowledge and behaviours. About halfway through coding, we began noticing certain regularities in the data which enabled us with some certainty to predict a given individual's likely responses to questions based on responses to previous questions. In the best tradition of grounded theory (Strauss and Corbin, 1990) a typology began to emerge. This seeks to relate sexual behaviour to attitudes. On the horizontal axis are sexual behaviours, ranging from an absence of sexual relationships at one end to multiple transitory contacts at the other. On the vertical axis are attitudes: at the one end those that are extremely conservative, and hostile to social differences, and at the other end liberal and proclaiming of respect for individual choices.

Respondent Type A, the 'conformist', combines conservative sexual behaviour with conservative attitudes. There has rarely been sexual education in the family of origin, and self-ascribed sexuality, if it is verbalized at all, is merely described as 'normal' in a fairly biological sense. Female virginity at marriage and the fidelity of one's wife are important, the latter in our Mediterranean sample being linked to a sense of honour rather than a conceptualization of relationship.

This person has little knowledge about HIV/AIDS, and either believes himself or herself to be at little personal risk, or, alternatively, as at great risk of infection

Figure 2 *Sexual Behaviour Related to Attitude*

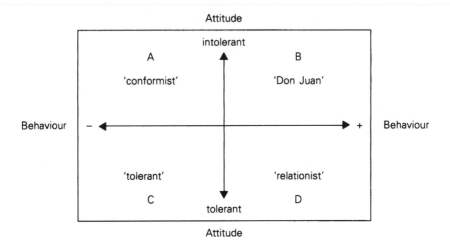

through dirty drinking glasses or insect bites, for example. Protective behaviours are either absent, or take place at the insistence of the other partner, such as on an occasional visit to a sex worker, for example. There is a marked attitude of rejection toward all people who might be considered 'different', including anyone affected by HIV unless that person is a family member.

Type B, the 'Don Juan', or the 'intolerant', has the same conservative attitudes, but has a sex life involving numerous partners; we have also on occasion called him (there are no women in this group) the 'macho'. He generally received his sex education from older comrades. Despite numerous transitory partners he never uses condoms. One 25-year-old, for example, explained that although there is a theoretical risk 'for a macho like me', in fact he is at little personal risk since he always checks the body odour of a potential partner, and in addition he knows who else she has been with. His HIV/AIDS knowledge is confused, and in fact he really prefers not to know anything.

Type C, the 'tolerant', has liberal attitudes but conservative sexual behaviour, often because of a conception of fidelity based on confidence in a relationship. He or she (the women in the sample tend to concentrate in this category) generally received sex education in the family of origin. HIV/AIDS knowledge is relatively good, as is an estimation of personal risk; protective behaviours therefore tend to be appropriate. The following male respondent is typical of this category:

> I respect everybody: prostitutes, addicts, I don't go to them myself, or smoke, or go with homosexuals. Since I am a Latin man, with hot blood, I like women a lot, but since I am married and I love the wife I have, I don't search any further. I've heard about a test for AIDS, I think it's free but I've never taken it. I have a friend who's homosexual who takes it from time to time . . . I think it would be important to know more about AIDS, how it's transmitted and how it's treated.

Type D, the 'relationist', combines liberal attitudes and numerous transitory sexual relationships, with an emphasis on the relationship aspect. Attitudes tend markedly towards respect for the choices of others, and towards solidarity. This combination of feeling was always associated with protective behaviour. As one such respondent put it:

> I always use a condom: it's better without, but I don't want to die. For me, the condom is part of my personal defense. I've used it systematically for the past four years. Even with somebody I know I always use it. . . . The concept of AIDS, it's not with hippies or punks or people who are poorly dressed . . . because the virus isn't going to choose people. . . .

In the sample studied, type A, the 'conformist', was the most frequently encountered (about twenty individuals), followed by type C, or the 'tolerant' (about fifteen people), then the two others in about equal proportions. It is, of course, type B who is at high risk, with a combination of risky behaviours, considerable incoherence in knowledge and a non-negligible dose of denial. While this particular typology, which again grew out of qualitative fieldwork, is in need of further testing and refinement, it worked reasonably well with the two populations studied. There is no a priori reason why its validity should be limited to Spanish and Portuguese seasonal workers in Switzerland.

Conclusions

Several conclusions can be reached at the end of this study of HIV/AIDS knowledge, attitudes and practices among seasonal migrant workers. First, the migrant workers in Switzerland studied here were much better informed about HIV/AIDS than predicted. On the other hand, transitory sexual relationships were most often unprotected. No evidence was found either that the incidence of transitory sexual relationships was higher among hotel personnel in a holiday resort, or, perhaps more apropos for AIDS prevention, that the migrant workers turned towards the 'grey market' of commercial sex workers possibly involved in injecting drug use. The study helped explain some of the dynamics of these various findings.

Second, from a methodological point of view, both qualitative and quantitative techniques were necessary. Semi-structured interviews provided a great deal of rich material, and the information gathered went far beyond what was necessary for a simple quantitative evaluation of HIV/AIDS knowledge and attitudes. Questions raised concerned broader issues such as migration and human relationships in general, including intimacy, power, honour and integration. However, such interviews were expensive, in terms of both time and effort; and it was often difficult for the research team to maintain its focus on the task at hand, an assessment of an HIV/AIDS prevention campaign. The paradox, and the difficulty, is that gathering such qualitative material is an essential prerequisite for the construction of a good tool for quantitative analysis. The language, and especially the cultural appropriateness and acceptability of questions, must be tested. Preparatory fieldwork is also essential to administering a questionnaire and knowing how to interpret the results.

Among the population studied here, the impersonal form of the standardized questionnaire was better adapted to gathering data concerning sexual behaviour and condom use. On the other hand, interview data and ethnographic fieldwork were important in allowing researchers to understand the dynamics of social relationships in the somewhat closed colony of the ski resort, and to assessing the possible magnitude, or lack thereof, of injecting drug use among a marginal population. Fieldwork alerted the researchers to the importance of attitudes as partial determinants of behaviour: we were able to propose a typology connecting attitudes to behaviour in a model to be tested in subsequent research. .

As a final step in the research process, feedback to the population studied is now underway, and Spanish- and Portuguese-speaking professionals have been engaged at local and national levels to develop and administer focused preventive programmes to the populations studied.

References

ANKRAH, M. (1989) 'AIDS: Methodological Problems in Studying Its Prevention and Spread', *Social Science and Medicine*, 29, 3, pp. 265–76.

BOLTANKSI, L. (1975) *Prime education et morale de classe*, Paris, Mouton.

DUBOIS-ARBER, F., LEHMANN, PH., HAUSSER, G. and GUTZWILLER, F. (1989) 'Evaluation des campagnes de prevention du SIDA en Suisse: Deuxième rapport de synthese', Lausanne, Institute universitaire de médécine sociale et preventive.

FLEURY, F., HAOUR-KNIPE, M. and OSPINA, S. (1991) 'Evaluation de la strategy de prevention du SIDA en Suisse', SIDA/Migration/Prevention, Dossier Portugais et Espagnol: 1989–90, Document 52.7, Lausanne, Institut universitaire de médécine sociale et preventive.

FRANKENBERG, R. (1986) 'Sickness as Cultural Performance: Drama, Trajectory and Pilgrimage. Root Metaphors and the Making Social of Disease', *International Journal of Health Services*, 16, 4, pp. 603–26.

HAOUR-KNIPE, M. (in preparation) 'Migrants and Travellers Group Final Report', European Community concerted action, Assessment of HIV/AIDS Preventive Strategies, Doc. 72, Lausanne, Institut universitaire de médécine sociale et preventive.

HERZLICH, C. and PIERRET, J. (1989) 'The Construction of a Social Phenomenon: AIDS in the French Press', *Social Science and Medicine*, 29, 11, pp. 1235–42.

HOMANS, H. and AGGLETON, P. (1988) 'Health education, HIV Infection and AIDS', in P. AGGLETON and H. HOMANS (Eds), *Social Aspects of AIDS*, Lewes, Falmer Press.

IPSO SOZIAL-UND UMFRAGEFORSCHUNG (1989) 'Enquête sur les comportements sexuels des jeunes adultes 17–30 ans', Lausanne, Institut universitaire de médécine sociale et preventive.

KAPLAN, H. (1989) 'Methodological Problems in the Study of Psychosocial Influences on the AIDS Process', *Social Science and Medicine*, 29, 3, pp. 227–92.

KLEINMAN, A. (1979) *Patients and Healers in the Context of Culture*, Berkeley, Calif., University of California Press.

MARTIN, J. and DEAN, L. (1990) 'Developing a Community Sample of Gay Men for an Epidemiologic Study of AIDS', *American Behavioral Scientist*, 33, 5, pp. 546–61.

MOERKERK, H., with AGGLETON, P. (1990) 'AIDS, 'Prevention Strategies in Europe: A Comparison and Critical Analysis', in P. AGGLETON, P. DAVIES and G. HART (Eds), *AIDS: Individual, Cultural and Policy Dimensions*, Lewes, Falmer Press.

OSPINA, S., HAOUR-KNIPE, M. and FLEURY, F. (1990) 'AIDS-Related Knowledge and Behaviour among Seasonal Workers in Switzerland', Paper presented at the Assessing AIDS Prevention conference, Montreux, Switzerland, 29 October–1 November 1990.

REGISTRE CENTRAL DES ÉTRANGERS (August, 1989) *Les étrangers en Suisse*, Berne, Office Fédéral de la Statistique.

SONTAG, S. (1989) *AIDS and Its Metaphors*, New York, Farrar, Straus and Giroux.

STEINAUER, J. (1980) *Le Saisonnier inexistant*, Geneva, Editions Que Faire?

STRAUSS, A. and CORBIN, J. (1990) *Basics of Qualitative Research: Grounded Theory Procedures and Techniques*, London, Sage.

STUTZ, T. and ZIMMERMANN, E. (1990) 'Aids Prevention in Switzerland', in S. WAYLING (Ed.), *Current Status of HIV/AIDS Prevention and Control Policies in the European Region: 1990 Update*, WHO Regional Office for Europe, EUR/ICP/GPA/ 079, 155–169.

VILLIEUMIER, M. (1987) *Immigrés et Refugiés en Suisse: Aperçu historique*, Zurich, Pro-Helvetia.

WISEMAN, T. (1989) 'Marginalized Groups and Health Education about HIV Infection and AIDS', in P. AGGLETON, P. DAVIES and G. HART (Eds), *AIDS: Social Representations, Social Practices*, Lewes, Falmer Press.

WORLD HEALTH ORGANISATION, GLOBAL PROGRAMME on AIDS (1988) Survey on AIDS-Related Knowledge, Attitudes, Beliefs and Practices Regarding HIV Infection and AIDS.

8 The Importance of Gay Community in the Prevention of HIV Transmission: A Study of Australian Men Who Have Sex with Men*

Susan Kippax, June Crawford, Bob Connell, Gary Dowsett, Lex Watson, Pam Rodden, Don Baxter and Rigmor Berg

In the context of the Acquired Immune Deficiency Syndrome (AIDS), gay sub-cultures have played and continue to play an active educative role. In Western countries, where gay men were among the first to suffer infection by the human immunodeficiency virus (HIV), gay communities took the lead in HIV prevention campaigns. For example, North American gay communities were among the first to suggest condoms to prevent the transmission of HIV in anal sex. In Australia, gay communities developed some of the most successful initiatives in Australian AIDS education. Dowsett (1989a, 1989b) has documented the importance of the gay community in Sydney as a source of information and educational material about HIV and 'safe sex'. In the United Kingdom, too, gay communities have taken a major role (Fitzpatrick, Boulton and Hart, 1989; Watney, 1990).

Among health educators and some researchers there is a recognition of the importance of gay communities to HIV prevention. In a discussion of comprehensive risk-reduction strategies for young people, DiClemente, Boyer and Mills (1987) pointed to the need for culturally relevant and sensitive educational material. Educational messages most likely to succeed are those which speak the language of the particular audience to which the messages are directed. Graham and Cates (1987) discussed the importance of initiatives taken by the leaders of the gay community in establishing an AIDS task force in Indiana; and Williams (1986) described the development of a strategy to encourage members of at-risk populations to assume leadership roles in education efforts to reduce HIV transmission.

---

* The Social Aspects of the Prevention of AIDS Project dedicates this chapter to Bruce Belcher and Gavin Murdoch, two of our field researchers who have since died of AIDS-related conditions.

Studies of sexual behaviour change among gay and bisexual men, however, do not always find a relationship between gay community attachment and change in sexual behaviour in response to HIV. Results of such studies are often complex. For example, in the United States Emmons *et al.* (1986) reported that although knowledge of HIV transmission was related to reported behaviour change, social norms were related only to a certain type of behaviour change, namely that concerning the number or type of one's sexual partners.

Given the beliefs of health educators and their commitment to community education programmes, the absence of a consistent research result is puzzling. Perhaps the reason for not finding the expected relationship between gay community and behaviour changes lies in the complexity of the meaning of gay community and in the difficulty of capturing that complexity in any survey measure. Also the assessment is complicated by the fact that there is usually considerable overlap between attachment to gay community and the AIDS epicentre. In their comparison of surveys conducted in the United States of America, DiClemente, Zorn and Temoshok (1987) noted that proximity to an AIDS epicentre has great saliency with respect to knowledge and attitudes about HIV/AIDS. In Australia, too, relationships have been found between place of residence and accuracy of information about safe sex practices among gay men (Kippax *et al.*, 1989, 1990). The same study also found relationships between place of residence and contact with the epidemic on the one hand, and change in sexual behaviour on the other (Connell *et al.*, 1989).

Gay men living in the Castro Street area in San Francisco and around Oxford Street in Sydney, both areas with a large gay population, are likely to have a high degree of contact with the epidemic. Men who live in these areas are very likely to have had friends who have died of AIDS and to know others who are infected with HIV. These men are also likely to have an attachment to gay community. Any change of sexual behaviour may therefore be related to all three variables; attachment to gay community, place of residence and contact with the epidemic.

The aims of the study reported in this chapter were to capture and quantify aspects of 'gay community' and to isolate the impact of gay community attachment on behaviour change. That is, it seeks to examine the effect of gay community attachment independently of the effect of closeness to the AIDS epicentre and of the effect of contact with the HIV epidemic.

Method and Analysis

The data on which this chapter is based derive from a large-scale research project, the Social Aspects of the Prevention of AIDS (SAPA), in which 535 gay and bisexual men in New South Wales (NSW) were interviewed. These men were recruited through gay organizations, by extensive media publicity and through networking; they comprise a volunteer non-clinical sample which was satisfactorily diverse except that working-class men were underrepresented. The interview took, on average, ninety minutes to complete. Men were asked about their sexual practices, social relationships, membership of and attachment to gay organizations and community, knowledge of and attitudes towards AIDS and safe sex, health practices and other issues. Typically, the interviews took place in respondents' homes. The majority of interviewers was gay men who had been trained in the project.

Fieldwork began in September 1986 and finished in March 1987 (for full details of sample and method see Connell *et al.*, 1987).

The analysis focused on developing gay identity and gay community scales, and on an examination of the relationship of these scales to social descriptor variables, such as age and class; and to those variables we called milieu variables, place of residence and the closeness to the epidemic measures. The impact of gay community on information and beliefs held about HIV and AIDS, on current sexual practice and on changes in sexual practices and the adoption of safe sex was also examined. This chapter limits itself to a description of the gay community scales and the impact of gay community on behaviour change.

Measures of Attachment of Gay Community

A sense of gay community is constituted in practices, both sexual and social. Gay community is produced in and has been transformed over time in gay bars and discos, at gay political meetings and rallies in 'beats' (places such as parks or public toilets where men may meet other men for sex), and in homes and social gatherings. It is constructed both in political and social activity and sexual practice. More recently, as Altman (1979, 1982) among others has noted, the HIV epidemic has reinforced an already strong sense of community among gay men.

At the same time, gay identity, identification of self as gay, has been transformed. It, too, is constructed in practice, both social and sexual, as well as in sexual preferences. As Weeks (1987) said of gay identity: 'For many in the modern world — especially the sexually marginal — it is an absolutely fundamental concept, offering a sense of personal unity, social location, and even at times a political commitment.'

Over sixty questions in the SAPA questionnaire concerned sexual identity, various forms of attachment to gay community and engagement in and identification with gay life. These questions were focused, in the main, on practice. There were questions about membership of gay organizations; further questions dealt with the places and venues where respondents sought contact of a social and sexual kind; and others dealt with whether the respondents patronized gay businesses, read gay newspapers and went to gay doctors. The responses to all these items were intercorrelated and factor analyzed. These analyses were examined with a view to constructing a number of gay identity and gay community scales.

Gay Identity

No scale measuring gay identity was found. The majority of men surveyed considered themselves gay (89 per cent) and believed that others knew of their gay identity (65 per cent). A small number did not identify as gay (7 per cent bisexual, 1 per cent heterosexual) and a somewhat larger number believed that others did not know of their sexual orientation (17 per cent heterosexual, 12 per cent don't know, 6 per cent bisexual).

Although no scale was found that gave a direct measure of gay identity, we were able to construct a reliable scale, the Gay Identity Disclosure scale (GID), which measures the degree to which men had disclosed their sexual identity to

Table 1 *Gay Identity Disclosure (GID) Scale*

Table 1   *Gay Identity Disclosure (GID) Scale*

Item	Item mean	Item-total correlation
1 Mother	0.63	0.58
2 Father	0.49	0.55
3 Other relative	0.66	0.46
4 Straight friends	0.90	0.31
5 Workmates	0.75	0.41
6 Neighbours	0.39	0.34
7 Other people	0.36	0.34

Note: Cronbach's alpha: 0.72.

others (parents, friends, workmates, neighbours). Almost all men in the sample had disclosed their identity to another gay man; most to someone not gay — friends and workmates being the most likely; and most had also disclosed to around four categories of persons (the mean scale score was 4.2). Gay Identity Disclosure is a measure of public commitment to one's gay identity.

Gay Community Involvement

No single factor of gay community attachment emerged. The exploratory factor analysis suggested the existence of at least three scales. We named these three scales 'Gay Community Involvement', 'Social Engagement in Gay Community' and 'Sexual Engagement in Gay Community'.

A number of intercorrelated items, indicating Gay Community Involvement (GCI), formed a reliable scale. This scale has twenty-one items and the item-total correlations are shown in Table 2. The scores ranged from 20 to 46 and were normally distributed around the mean scale score of 32.6 with a standard deviation of 5.2. Someone with a high score has a wide range of involvement in gay community: he would be likely to read gay newspapers, patronize gay shops and businesses, go to a gay-identified doctor, attend gay functions (sporting, political, social) and be a member of gay organizations (both social and AIDS-related). In essence, this scale measures the degree of men's 'immersion' in modern gay culture and politics.

Social Engagement Scale

Another ten items formed a scale which we identified as a measure of Social Engagement (SCE). The scores ranged from 9 to 23 with a mean of 19.0 and a standard deviation of 2.5. The distribution is skewed with the majoritty of men scoring between 20 and 23, that is, having a degree of social contact with other gay and bisexual men. Men with relatively high scores on this scale are likely to have many gay male friends. They are also likely to spend much of their free time with gay men, and much of their social contact takes place in gay bars, discos as well as private parties and meetings. These men's attachment is lived out as a

Table 2   *Gay Community Involvement (GCI) Scale*

Item		Item mean	Item-total r
1	Identifies with gay community (g.c.)	2.73	0.36
2	Goes to gay-identified doctor	2.10	0.32
3	Reads gay newspapers	2.46	0.36
4	Goes to g.c. sporting functions	1.27	0.30
5	Goes to g.c. political functions	1.24	0.41
6	Goes to g.c. social group functions	1.59	0.44
7	Goes to g.c. religious functions	1.13	0.23
8	Goes to g.c. counselling groups	1.24	0.39
9	Goes to g.c. AIDS-related groups	1.35	0.43
10	Goes to g.c. university/college groups	1.10	0.16
11	Member of g.c. organizations	1.67	0.59
12	Member of g.c. sporting club	1.15	0.29
13	Member of g.c. political group	1.26	0.43
14	Member of g.c. social group	1.48	0.48
15	Member of g.c. religious group	1.13	0.27
16	Member of g.c. counselling group	1.26	0.46
17	Member of g.c. AIDS-related group	1.32	0.50
18	Member of g.c. university/college group	1.15	0.26
19	Patronizes gay shops and businesses	1.87	0.40
20	Goes to gay films/theatre	2.12	0.43
21	Reads books with gay themes	1.96	0.43

Note: Cronbach's alpha: 0.81.

Table 3   *Social Engagement (SCE) Scale*

Item		Item mean	Item total r
1	Spends time with gay friends	3.50	0.50
2	Friends are gay men	1.58	0.45
3	Goes out with gay friends (g.f.)	1.96	0.40
4	Goes out with g.f. to bars	1.79	0.40
5	Goes out with g.f. to theatre/films	1.89	0.41
6	Goes out with g.f. to discos/dances	1.72	0.44
7	Goes out with g.f. to private parties	1.89	0.47
8	Goes out with g.f. to bookshops	1.26	0.21
9	Goes out with g.f. to pool/beach	1.75	0.38
10	Goes out with g.f. to meetings	1.71	0.28

Note: Cronbach's alpha: 0.71.

social engagement with gay community. The items and the item-total correlations are shown in Table 3.

Sexual Engagement Scale

A third scale, which we called the Sexual Engagement scale (SXE), was made up of nineteen items which measure the number of casual partners and the frequency of casual sex, as well as men's use of sex venues such as saunas and beats to find partners, both social and sexual. The items and the item-total correlations are

Table 4   Sexual Engagement (SXE) Scale

Item		Item mean	Item total r
1	No casual partners last six months	1.80	0.62
2	Frequency of casual sex	0.85	0.59
3	Uses gay video pornography	1.86	0.19
4	Seeks sexual partners at bars	1.66	0.43
5	Seeks sexual partners at saunas	1.39	0.51
6	Seeks sexual partners at discos	1.59	0.38
7	Seeks sexual partners at parties	1.68	0.35
8	Seeks sexual partners at beats	1.37	0.51
9	Seeks sexual partners at bookshops	1.13	0.34
10	Seeks sexual partners at sex cinema	1.04	0.28
11	Seeks male prostitutes	1.04	0.22
12	Seeks sexual partners at gym	1.16	0.21
13	Seeks sexual partners at pool/beach	1.43	0.37
14	Seeks social contact at saunas	1.19	0.39
15	Seeks social contact at beats	1.12	0.29
16	Seeks social contact at sex cinema	1.03	0.17
17	Seeks social contact at wall*	1.02	0.14
18	Uses venues for sex with casual partner	1.69	0.63
19	Uses venues for sex with regular partner	1.15	0.21

Notes: Cronbach's alpha: 0.79.
* A meeting place for young male prostitutes.

Table 5   Relationship between Gay Identity Disclosure and Community Attachment Scales

Correlations between the scales

	Gay Identity Disclosure	Gay Community Involvement	Social Engagement	Sexual Engagement
GID	1.00	0.34*	0.25*	0.05
GCI		1.00	0.48*	0.17*
SCE			1.00	0.22*
SXE				1.00

Note: * p < 0.001.

shown in Table 4. The scores on this table range from 17 to 40 with a mean scale score of 25.2 and a standard deviation of 4.5. The distribution was slightly negatively skewed: most men had some degree of sexual engagement in gay community, but some, approximately 20 per cent had little sexual engagement in gay community as measured by this scale.

Thus the analysis revealed three forms of attachment to gay community, cultural/political, social and sexual, and a measure of public commitment as captured by the Gay Identity Disclosure scale. All four measures were intercorrelated, indicating that attachment to gay community is lived out in a number of overlapping ways. Although the high correlation between the community involvement and social engagement scales suggested the possibility of a single scale, the content of the two sets of items is sufficiently different to keep them separate (see Table 5). The relatively small correlations between the Sexual Engagement scale and the other two gay community attachment scales indicated that men who engage in casual sex and seek sexual partners in a variety of venues are not necessarily socially or culturally/politically involved in gay community.

There were strong positive correlations between the Gay Identity Disclosure scale and both the Gay Community Involvement and Social Engagement scales, but no relationship between it and the Sexual Engagement scale was found. These data indicated a stronger public commitment to gay community among the men whose attachment is either cultural/political or social as opposed to sexual. Also indicated is that some men who are sexually engaged with other men have kept this aspect of their life hidden from their family friends and social networks. In gay community parlance, these men might be described as being 'in the closet'. This does not necessarily mean that these men are uncomfortable about their gay identity or sexual preference. Men who are sexually engaged in gay community but who have told few others of their sexual interests may be perfectly at home with their sexuality, but deem it unnecessary or perhaps unsafe to tell others.

Social Descriptor Variables in Relation to Gay Community

Further analysis revealed that these four scales were related to a number of social descriptor variables such as age, education and, very importantly, region or place of residence. While men from all social backgrounds and classes participate in the social and sexual offerings of gay community life, cultural and political involvement is limited to middle-class men. The Gay Community Involvement scale is the only scale to show significant and positive relationships with a number of social descriptor or demographic variables — education, occupational status and income. It may be that these middle-class men were and continue to be a substantial part of the gay liberation movement.

Age was related to the two engagement scales. There was more active sexual engagement in gay community among men aged 30 years and older and less social engagement among men aged 39 and over. There is a slight tendency among the young to favour a social rather than a sexual engagement in gay community life, perhaps as one result of the impact of HIV.

These data confirmed our initial interpretation: that there are three forms of gay community attachment captured by our data. This does not mean that there are three types of gay man. Rather, the data indicated that there are men whose attachment to gay community is expressed in all three ways outlined below, others for whom attachment is constituted in only one or two of these forms and others for whom any form of attachment is minimal.

These three forms of attachment may be characterized in the following ways: the first as measured on the GCI scale is primarily a cultural and political involvement in gay community. Men with a strong gay community involvement are likely to be middle-class professional men who are confident in their identity and have disclosed it to many: their relatives, friends, workmates and neighbours.

The second takes the form of a social engagement, as measured by the SCE scale. Those whose attachment is social are younger but in terms of class are a far more heterogeneous group than those with a cultural and political involvement. Like the men with a cultural and political involvement, these socially attached men identify as gay and are likely to disclose their identity to others. Their gay

Table 6   Gay Community Attachment and Identity Disclosure Scale Mean Scores on Social Descriptor Variables

	Scale Means			
	GCI	SCE	SXE	GID
Age:				
< 19	31.27	19.05	24.32	3.45
20–29	32.25	19.38	24.35	4.18
30–39	32.86	19.13	26.09	4.46
40–49	32.96	18.38	25.25	3.78
50+	33.06	17.96	24.96	3.50
	NS	***	***	*
National origin:	NS	NS	NS	NS
Religion:				
Agnostic	33.30	19.12	24.95	4.52
Protestant	32.35	19.19	25.39	3.98
Catholic	32.01	18.78	25.24	3.59
Other	31.16	18.77	25.42	4.04
	*	NS	NS	***
Education:				
Up to Year 11	30.99	18.80	25.60	3.86
Years 11 and 12	32.51	19.26	25.28	4.21
Post-secondary	31.70	18.94	25.01	4.35
Higher education	33.75	19.07	24.95	4.30
	***	NS	NS	NS
Occupation:				
Managerial/professional	33.38	19.18	25.31	4.38
Paraprofessional	32.57	19.05	24.80	3.97
Sales/unskilled	31.56	18.95	26.22	4.05
	*	NS	NS	NS
Income:				
< 12,000	31.27	18.70	24.55	4.32
12,001–18,000	32.76	19.22	25.16	4.09
18,001–26,000	33.08	19.30	25.40	4.18
26,001 +	33.04	19.00	25.47	4.20
	*	NS	NS	NS
Labour force status:	NS	NS	NS	NS

Notes: * $p < 0.05$;
** $p < 0.01$;
*** $p < 0.005$.

identity is constituted in their friendships and their leisure pursuits, but not necessarily in their membership of gay organizations.

The third form of attachment is characterized by sexual engagement. Although those whose engagement is sexual are likely to be older than men whose attachment is social, they come from all walks of life. Further, although they are less likely than men with a cultural and political involvement or social engagement in gay community to have disclosed their sexual preference to others, they are just as likely to identify themselves as gay. It is as though their identity is constituted in sexual rather than social or cultural practices, even though, for many, their sexual practices are separate from the rest of their lives.

Table 7   Mean Gay Community and Contact with the Epidemic Scores by Locale

| Locale | Mean scale scores | | | | |
	GCI	SCE	SXE	GID	CE
Inner Sydney	33.42	19.53	25.59	4.53	1.75
North Suburbs	32.41	18.81	25.22	4.09	1.19
Outer Sydney	31.05	18.55	24.98	3.22	0.91
X-Metropolitan NSW	30.19	18.15	24.19	4.19	1.06
Canberra	33.03	19.15	24.00	3.38	0.75
	***	***	NS	***	***

Note: *** p < 0.001.

Gay Community, Locale and Contact with HIV

We now turn to assess the impact of gay attachment on behaviour change. To do this, however, it is first necessary to examine the relationship between such measures of attachment and variable which measure degree of contact with the epidemic and place of residence.

Place of residence is an important concept with regard to gay community and HIV transmission. Oxford Street, the public focus of much gay activity in Sydney, and the inner-city suburbs are the suburbs in which many gay men choose to live (121 men (22.6 per cent) in the sample had moved to Sydney in the five years prior to the survey, and 85 per cent of these men had moved to the inner-Sydney suburbs). These areas house many of the gay bars, discos, saunas, business and meeting places. A variable we called 'locale' was created to assess place of residence. The five locales are Inner Sydney, which takes in Oxford Street, the eastern suburbs of Sydney and the inner city; Northern Suburbs; Outer Sydney, which takes in the southern, the western, and south-western suburbs; Extra-metropolitan NSW, both towns and centres; and Canberra.

Locale is also important because of claims that changes in sexual practice have occurred *because* of gay men's contact with the epidemic. The epicentre of HIV/AIDS is identified with the Oxford Street and inner-Sydney area. Men who live in this area are likely to have had more contact with the epidemic, as well as more contact with gay community responses to HIV/AIDS, than men who live in the outer suburbs and outside Sydney. A variable to assess degree of contact with the epidemic (CE) was developed from three items: knowing anyone with AIDS, caring or nursing people with AIDS, and knowing anyone who has died of AIDS (see Connell *et al.*, 1989). The relationships between contact with the epidemic and men's HIV test status (untested, negative and positive) and gay community attachment were also examined.

Locale was significantly associated with a cultural/political involvement and social engagement in gay community as well as disclosure of gay identity (see Table 7). While men in Inner Sydney had the strongest attachments to gay community and men in Outer Sydney and in Extra-metropolitan NSW were least likely to be socially engaged with or involved in gay community, men in all locales had some form of attachment to gay community. That is, although the Inner Sydney locale may be better supplied with bars, discos and saunas, all

Table 8 Mean Gay Community and Contact with the Epidemic Scores by Test Status

Test status			Mean scale scores		
	GCI	SCE	SXE	GID	CE
Untested	31.1	18.5	24.2	3.7	1.2
Test seropositive	33.0	19.2	25.4	4.4	1.5
Test seronegative	34.0	19.6	26.5	4.5	1.8
	***	***	***	***	***

Note: *** $p < 0.001$.

locales are able to offer meeting places for social, cultural/political and sexual contact. The most striking aspect of Table 7, however, is that unlike the other gay community attachment measures, men's sexual engagement with gay community is unrelated to place of residence.

Contact with Epidemic/HIV Test Status

Contact with the epidemic was, as predicted, greatest for those men who live in Inner Sydney, and proportionately more of these Inner Sydney men had been tested than in any other locale (73.4 per cent compared with 51.8 per cent in Extra-metropolitan NSW and 55.5 per cent in Outer Sydney). Test status was also significantly related to the measures of gay community attachment and gay identity disclosure (see Table 8). Those men with the strongest attachment to gay community and those who were more likely to have disclosed their identity were more likely to have been tested than not. Note, however, that the outcome of the test was unrelated to these gay community measures.

Summary of Scales and Relationship with Other Measures

Locale and Contact with the Epidemic were far more closely related to gay community attachment than the social descriptor variables discussed above. The social descriptors were, with the exception of the class-related variables and age, unrelated to gay community, whereas locale, contact with epidemic and test status (tested versus untested) were very closely related.

Respondents who lived in Inner Sydney embraced gay life. Of these, men who are well educated were likely to have a strong sense of gay community involvement, while the young were likely to have a social engagement with gay community. Men who live in Inner Sydney were also likely to have disclosed their identity to most others; they appeared confident in their gay identity. These men were also the men with the greatest contact with the epidemic.

Men who live in other locales, however, were also attached to gay community, but in different ways. Some were culturally and politically involved and others were socially engaged. Locale may limit the *ways* these forms of attachment are lived but it does not appear to limit the attachment itself. Sexual engagement is, however, unaffected by locale: it was independent of locale and most of the social descriptors.

Thus the three forms of gay community attachment identified and discussed earlier in this chapter were closely related to locale, and, in turn, to contact with the epidemic. This was especially true for the forms of gay community attachment captured by the Gay Community Involvement scale and the Social Engagement scale. Inner Sydney, the Northern Suburbs and Canberra offer a greater range of ways to attach oneself to gay community. It is of interest to note, however, that the men who live in the Extra-metropolitan NSW and the Inner Sydney locales were more likely to have disclosed their identity to others. Being gay takes many forms — social, sexual and cultural/political — and is lived out in a variety of ways, publicly and privately, in different places.

Changes in Sexual Behaviour

The remainder of this chapter examines the impact of the gay community variables, as well as locale and Contact with the Epidemic, on changes in sexual behaviour. The regression analyses also included measures of forms of sexual practice (Connell and Kippax, 1990), measures of information and knowledge (Kippax *et al.*, 1990), and relationships between these (Connell *et al.*, 1989, 1990). A detailed statistical examination is found in Crawford, Kippax and Dowsett (1990).

Gay Community and Change in Behaviour

Change in behaviour was measured by two scales. The first scale, Adopting Safe Sex (AS), measures actual changes in sexual behaviour such as the use of condoms and the foregoing of fisting. The second scale, Relationship Change (RC), measures changes such as a move to monogamy or the reduction of the number of casual sexual partners.

The variables included in the multiple regression were those which were significant in univariate analyses. These were the social descriptor variables, age and education; the milieu variables, locale, Contact with the Epidemic, HIV test status; three gay community attachment scales, GCI, SCE, SXE; and the knowledge scales, KSS, KUS, GI and PA. The sexual practice scales, OTP, EAP and IEP, as well as relationship status were also included. The dependent variables were sexual behaviour change (AS) and relationship change (RC).

Sexual Behaviour Change

The variables which contributed most to sexual behaviour change (AS) were two of the gay community attachment scales: sexual engagement and social engagement; and locale. Another variable of some importance was knowledge of 'unsafe' sex. The nature of sexual relationship and sexual practice were also implicated, but these may be simply functions of change as well as predictors of it (see Table 9).

In the full model, the variables accounted for 23.2 per cent of the variance in sexual behaviour change. The social descriptor variables when fitted alone accounted for 1.5 per cent, the milieu variables for 15.2 per cent and the knowledge

Table 9   Regression Model: Behaviour Change

| Variable | Full model | | | Reduced model | | | | % var fit last |
| | r | R^2 (%) | % var fit last | Regression coefficients | | t | p | |
				Raw	Standard			
Age	−.033	0.1	0.3					
Education	.111	1.2	0.9	.193	.113	2.79	.005	1.2
None				.460	.224	1.56	.119	
Monogamous				−.650	−.315	−2.50	.013	
Several		7.8	2.6	.715	.348	2.07	.039	2.8
Regular plus (compared with casual only				.064	.031	0.27	.784	
SXE	.337	11.3	2.7	.098	.215	4.35	.000	2.9
SCE	.196	3.8	0.4	.081	.097	2.25	.025	1.0
GCI	.185	3.4	0.1					
North Suburbs				.310	.151	0.99	.323	
Outer Sydney				−.183	−.089	−0.69	.493	
X-metropolitan		3.4	0.7	−.480	−.234	−1.96	.050	0.9
Canberra (compared with Inner Sydney)				−.076	−.037	−0.24	.811	
CE	.162	2.6	0.5	.121	.063	1.44	.150	0.1
KSS	.016	0.0	0.0					
KUS	.119	1.4	1.4	.113	.123	3.09	.002	1.4
KSP	.028	0.1	0.1					
GI	.136	1.8	0.5					
PA	.115	1.3	0.2					
Positive				.518	.253	1.91	.057	
Negative (compared with untested)		1.7	0.5	.164	.080	0.84	.402	0.6
IEP	.036	0.1	0.6	−.133	−.096	−2.25	.025	0.6
EAP	.092	0.8	0.0					
OTP	.161	2.6	0.7	.194	.134	2.89	.004	1.0
	R^2 = 23.05%			R^2 = 21.8%				

variables for 5.8 per cent. The milieu and community attachment variables were clearly the most important set. What the analysis showed is that locale and attachment to gay community, particularly sexual engagement and, to a lesser extent, social engagement, are most important for change in sexual behaviour. The greater the engagement, the greater the change.

An accurate knowledge of 'unsafe' sexual practice contributed to a change to 'safe' sexual behaviour. Education contributed a small amount to change; men with more years of education were more likely to have changed their practice in the direction of 'safe' sex than men with fewer years of education. As might be expected, those in monogamous relationships had changed least, while those in several relationships had changed most. Also men who engaged in a wide variety of oral and tactile sexual practices had changed most. It is likely that the significant relationships between sexual relationship status and sexual practice, on the one hand, and change in sexual practice, on the other, were a result of a move to these 'safe' sexual practices by the men surveyed rather than predictors of that change.

The importance of locale was indicated by the finding that those who live in Extra-metropolitan NSW have changed least when compared with men who live in Inner Sydney. This relationship holds over and above gay community attachment. On the other hand, Contact with the Epidemic is not important once the gay community attachment variables and locale variables are taken into account. Gay community attachment and locale are important explanatory concepts over and above their relationship with Contact with the Epidemic.

Relationship Change

A similar regression analysis was carried out with relationship change as the dependent variable. The reduced model showed that knowledge of 'safe' sex and locale were important variables with regard to relationship change, as was education level. Measures of attachment to gay community were not strongly related to relationship change; sexual engagement in gay community was marginally significant; those with the lowest sexual engagement were the most likely to change the nature of their relationships (see Table 10). This is the reverse of the relationship which held between the adoption of safe sex and sexual engagement in gay community.

The full model accounted for 14.2 per cent of the variance and the reduced model for 10.4 per cent (12.1 per cent if sexual relationship status is included). The analysis indicated that men with little accurate knowledge of 'safe' sex and with little education were more likely to change their relationship status than others. It is almost as though they change their relationship status because they are not sure which sexual practices are 'safe'. Gay community attachment was of little importance, while locale had some impact on relationship change. Men in Extra-metropolitan NSW and men in the Northern Suburbs, when compared with men in Inner Sydney, were most likely to have changed their sexual relationships towards monogamy and celibacy.

Summary of Behaviour Change

In general, gay community attachment and locale are important predictors of change. These data confirm the importance of informed social support. It appears that educators who stress the need to address communities from the point of view of the communities themselves are correct. Gay community and locale are also implicated in the relationship between knowledge and change. Knowledge of 'safe' sex, something that to some extent only the gay communities dealt with in their media and educational campaigns, is also implicated in change. Men who do not know what is 'safe' sex are the ones most likely to change their relationship status.

Contact with the epidemic is important, but its impact on change is mediated by gay community attachment. If there is no gay community attachment, then contact with the epidemic is a contributor towards sexual behaviour change.

Table 10   Regression Model: Relationship Change

Variable	Full model			Reduced model				% var fit last
	r	R² (%)	% var fit last	Regression coefficients Raw	Standard	t	p	
Age	.011	0.0	0.0					
Education	–.132	1.7	0.9	–.257	–.115	–2.73	.007	1.3
None Monogamous Several Regular plus (compared with casual only		2.5	0.9					
SXE	–.070	0.5	0.8	–048	–.080	–1.92	.055	0.6
SCE	–.043	0.2	0.0					
GCI	–.059	0.3	0.0					
North Suburbs				.906	.336	2.15	.032	
Outer Sydney				.065	.024	0.18	.865	
X-metropolitan			2.2	.967	.358	2.95	.003	2.8
Canberra				–.404	–.150	–0.94	.346	
(compared with Inner Sydney)								
CE	.023	0.1	0.2					
KSS	–.244	6.0	1.5	–.170	–.207	–4.89	.000	4.1
KUS	.155	2.4	0.1					
KSP	–.133	1.8	0.2					
GI	.106	1.1	0.0					
PA	–.083	0.7	0.1					
Positive Negative (compared with untested)		0.7	0.9					
IEP	.027	0.1	0.1					
EAP	.043	0.2	0.3					
OTP	–.067	0.4	0.4					

R² = 14.2%

R² = 10.4%
Note: if sexual relationships included, SXE is not significant and reduced model, R² = 12.1%

However, if attachment to gay community is present, this variable adds little by way of a contribution to change. The test result is, in general, unimportant.

Conclusions

Despite evidence to the contrary from other studies, this study points to the importance of gay community attachment to sexual behaviour change and to a lesser extent relationship change. The sexually confident, well-educated gay men who live in Sydney or Canberra who are sexually and socially engaged with gay community, and who are well informed about 'safe' and 'unsafe' sex are more likely to have changed their sexual behaviour than gay men who are not attached to gay community, who live in extra-metropolitan NSW, who have had little contact with the epidemic and are unsure of what is 'safe'. This latter group is to some degree more likely than the former to change the nature of their sexual relationships to protect themselves from HIV infection. It is important to note, however, that there are not two separate identifiable groups of men: one group who change their sexual behaviour; the other who change the nature of their relationships. Some men have changed both their sexual practice and the nature of their relationships, others have changed little with regard to either, and yet other men have modified aspects of both their sexual behaviour and their relationships (Connell *et al.*, 1989). Both strategies involve risk; 'safe' sex may be difficult to sustain over a period of time, and relationship changes do not necessarily protect one from infection. With regard to the latter point, recent figures suggest that there is an increase in the number of men in regular relationships who are becoming infected (Tindall *et al.*, 1989).

It is evident that health promotion campaigns should continue to be informed by gay communities. It also seems that the men who are most at risk are those who are not reached by gay community campaigns. Men who, for whatever reason, are separate from any form of attachment to gay community need special attention. Many of these men appear not to be sure about the sexual practices in which they can safely engage with virtually no risk of HIV infection. What these data indicate is the importance of support from similar others. This is not surprising given that sexual behaviour takes place *between* two or more people, an often overlooked fact in the HIV/AIDS literature.

In general, men in contact with others, via attachment to gay community — sexual, social or cultural/political — are most likely to have changed their sexual practice. They have the informed social support necessary to modify their behaviour. Men who are isolated from others like themselves and are unattached to gay community in any form are those least likely to change. Some of these 'unattached' men have changed because of their contact with the epidemic; others have not. To protect themselves, some of them appear to have changed the nature of their sexual relationships — to have moved to monogamy or celibacy. Those most likely to have made these moves are those who live outside, away from the public centres of gay community.

This raises a question about the continued coyness and lack of clarity with respect to male-to-male sex and HIV transmission in our national AIDS education campaign. Gay community education efforts work; but they only reach so far beyond the local gay communities, and they rely on some form of attachment to gay community. Either gay community education needs to be resourced sufficiently and charged with the responsibility of reaching out far beyond its current focus; or mainstream education is going to have to bite the bullet and become more explicit and determined to reach all men who have sex with men.

Acknowledgments

We acknowledge grants from the New South Wales and Commonwealth Department of Health and the Macquarie University Research Grants Committee. We wish to thank all those who took part in the study, respondents and interviewers.

References

ALTMAN, D. (1979) *Coming Out in the Seventies*, Sydney, Wild and Woolley.

ALTMAN, D. (1982) *The Homosexualisation of America, the Americanization of the Homosexual*, New York, St Martin's Press.

CONNELL, R.W. and KIPPAX, S. (1990) 'Sexuality in the AIDS Crisis: Patterns of Sexual Practice and Pleasure in a Sample of Australian Gay and Bisexual Men', *The Journal of Sex Research*, 27, 2, pp. 1–32.

CONNELL, R.W., CRAWFORD, J., KIPPAX, S., DOWSETT, G.W., BOND, G., BAXTER, D., BERG, R. and WATSON, L. (1987) 'Method and Sample, Social Aspects of the Prevention of AIDS, Study A Report No. 1', Sydney, Macquarie University School of Behavioural Sciences.

CONNELL, R.W., CRAWFORD, J., KIPPAX, S., DOWSETT, G.W., BAXTER, D., WATSON, L. and BERG, R. (1989) 'Facing the Epidemic: Changes in the Sexual Lives of Gay and Bisexual Men in Australia and their implication for AIDS Prevention Strategies, *Social Problems*, 36, 4, pp. 384–402.

CONNELL, R.W., CRAWFORD, J., DOWSETT, G.W., KIPPAX, S., SINNOTT, V., RODDEN, P., BERG, R., BAXTER, D. and WATSON, L. (1990) 'Danger and Context: Unsafe Anal Sexual Practice among Homosexual and Bisexual Men', *Australian and New Zealand Journal of Sociology*, 26, 2, pp. 187–208.

CRAWFORD, J., KIPPAX, S. and DOWSETT, G.W. (1990) 'The Role of Contact with the HIV/AIDS Epidemic in Determining Behaviour Change in a Sample of Homosexual and Bisexual Men', in P.J. SOLOMAN, C. FAZEKAS DE ST GROTH and S.R. WILSON (Eds), *Projections of Acquired Immune Deficiency Syndrome in Australia Using Data to the End of September 1989*, Working Papers 16, 89–91. National Centre for Epidemiology and Population Health.

DiCLEMENTE, R.J., BOYER, C.B. and MILLS, S.J. (1987) 'Prevention of AIDS among Adolescents: Strategies for the Development of Comprehensive Risk-reduction Health Education Programs', *Health Education Research*, 2, 3, pp. 287–91.

DiCLEMENTE, R.J., ZORN, J. and TEMOSHOK, L. (1987) 'The Association of Gender, Ethnicity and Length of Residence in the Bay Area to Adolescents' Knowledge and Attitudes about Acquired Immune Deficiency Syndrome', *Journal of Applied Social Psychology*, 17, 3, pp. 216–30.

DOWSETT, G.W. (1989a) '"You'll Never Forget the Feeling of Safe Sex!": AIDS Prevention strategies for Gay and Bisexual Men in Sydney, Australia', Paper presented at the World Health Organisation Workshop on AIDS Health Promotion Activities Directed towards Gay and Bisexual Men, Geneva, 29–31 May.

DOWSETT, G.W. (1989b) 'Reaching Men Who Have Sex with Men in Australia', Paper presented at the World Health Organisation Second International Symposium on AIDS Information and Education, Yaoundé, Cameroon, 22–26 October.

EMMONS, C.A., JOSEPH, J.G., KESSLER, R.C., WORTMAN, C.B., MONTGOMERY, S. and OSTROW, D. (1986) 'Psychological Predictors of Reported Behaviour Change in Homosexual Men at Risk for AIDS', *Health Education Quarterly*, 13, 4, pp. 331–45.

FITZPATRICK, R., BOULTON, M. and HART, G. (1989) 'Gay Men's Sexual Behaviour in Response to AIDS: Insights and Problems', in P. AGGLETON, P. DAVIES and G. HART (Eds), *AIDS: Social Representations, Social Practices*, Lewes Falmer Press.

GRAHAM, L. and CATES, J.A. (1987) 'AIDS: Developing a Primary Health Care Task Force', *Journal of Psychosocial Nursing and Mental Health Services*, 25, 12, pp. 21–5.

KIPPAX, S., BOND, G., SINNOTT, V., CRAWFORD, J., DOWSETT, G.W., BAXTER, D., BERG, R., CONNELL, R.W. and WATSON, L. (1989) 'Regional Differences in the Responses of Gay and Bisexual Men to AIDS: The Australian Capital Territory, Social Aspects of the Prevention of AIDS, Study A Report No. 4, Sydney, Macquarie University, School of Behavioural Sciences.

KIPPAX, S., CRAWFORD, J., BOND, G., SINNOTT, V., BAXTER, D., BERG, R., CONNELL, R.W., DOWSETT, G.W. and WATSON, L. (1990) 'Information about AIDS: The Accuracy of Knowledge Possessed by Gay and Bisexual Men', *Australian Journal of Social Issues*, 25, 3, pp. 199–219.

TINDALL, B., SWANSON, C., DONOVAN, B. and COOPER, D.A. (1989) 'Sexual Practices and Condom Usage in a Cohort of Homosexual Men in Relation to Human Immunodeficiency Virus Status', *Medical Journal of Australia*, 151, pp. 318–22.

WATNEY, S. (1990) 'Safer Sex as Community Practice', in P. AGGLETON, P. DAVIES and G. HART (Eds), *AIDS: Individual, Cultural and Policy Dimensions*, Lewes, Falmer Press.

WEEKS, J. (1987) 'Questions of Identity', in P. CAPLAN (Ed.), *The Cultural Construction of Sexuality*, London, Tavistock.

WILLIAMS, L.S. (1986) 'AIDS Risk Reduction: A Community Health Education Intervention for Minority High Risk Group Members', *Health Education Quarterly*, 13, 4, pp. 407–21.

9 Alcohol Use and Unsafe Sexual Behaviour: Any Connection?

Peter Weatherburn and Project SIGMA[1]

Drinke, Sir, is a greater prouoker of three things, . . . Nofe painting, Sleepe, and Vrine. Lecherie, Sir, it prouokes, it unprouokes: it prouokes the defire but it takes away the performance. Therefore, much Drinke may be faid to be an Equiuocator with Lecherie: it makes him and it marres him, it fets him on and it takes him off; it perfuades him and difheartens him; makes him ftand too, and not ftand too: in conclusion, equiuocates him in a Sleepe, and giuing him the Lye, leaues him. (Macbeth II, iii)

The assertion that there is an association between 'risky' sexual behaviour and alcohol and/or drug use (more commonly and revealingly termed 'abuse' or 'misuse') has become commonplace (Ostrow, 1986; Stall *et al.*, 1986; Stall, 1987; Valdisserri *et al.*, 1988; Hingson *et al.*, 1990; Goldbeck and Molgaard, 1990), and indeed seems to have become such an entrenched part of accepted knowledge that Goldbeck and Molgaard (1990, p. 1) can state: 'It is widely accepted that alcohol consumption *during sexual activity* is associated with increased risk of [AIDS] through the practice of risky sexual behaviors which increase the chance of exposure to HIV' [emphasis added].

Widely accepted it may be, but *proven* the link most certainly is not. Quite apart from the assumption that alcohol use is relatively uncommon during sex but relatively common before or after it, this chapter contends that the link is asserted and not proven; that the evidence is at best contradictory and that this assertion is informed by a puritanical moral agenda: At best, the current orthodoxy provides a partial explanation of the link between alcohol use, unsafe sex and HIV. At worst, it is costly, misguided and profoundly short-sighted. In fact, on the basis of the data reported here, we prefer Shakespeare's account to that of many contemporary researchers.

In this chapter we critically examine some of the literature on alcohol use and unsafe sexual behaviour and discuss the assumptions underlying recent research in this field. Empirical and qualitative data from Project SIGMA are used to elucidate the complex nature of the relationship.

The Orthodox Account of Alcohol Use and 'Risky' Sex

Before some of the assumptions that underpin current research agendas are discussed, it is important to state that our interest in this chapter is focused only on alcohol. Unfortunately, some of the recent literature fails to distinguish between different psychoactive drugs — of which alcohol is the most commonly used. Instead, it refers to psychoactive drugs and alcohol in the same sentence as if there were no difference in terms of the reasons for their use, the social contexts and the physical, psychological and behavioural effects of their consumption. This is unacceptable.

Some six years ago Ostrow (1986, p. 15) of the American Multicentre AIDS Cohort Study (MACS) claimed:

> There are significant barriers, among health professionals and the general public, to recognizing the role that drugs and alcohol may play in AIDS and the need to identify drug and alcohol problems in persons who have the active disease or are carrying the virus. Epidemiological data conclusively show the close interrelation between drug abuse, sexual activity, and transmission of infection.

It should be noted that the first sentence makes a point about the effects of 'drugs and alcohol' on people with HIV, while the second makes an assertion about transmission. As highlighted above, these are quite separate issues. Nevertheless, his claim that data showed 'conclusively' the interrelation between drug 'abuse', sex and HIV transmission is at best debatable, but it did much to set the narrow and, we will argue, misguided research agenda in this field. Six years on, conclusive data still do not exist, and the search for such 'strong interrelations' is misguided, naïve and counter-productive. (Ostrow, 1986, p. 18) went on to claim:

> . . . [we] are clearly establishing an association between drug and alcohol abuse in a subpopulation of gay men and unsafe sexual practices known to transmit AIDS infection [sic]. This association becomes even more powerful the more proximal the period of reported drug use is to sexual behavior that is considered unsafe. The correlations between receptive anal intercourse, the number of different sexual partners, and the use of various psychoactive substances are extremely high.

While he was being careful to acknowledge that there was no proof of an 'informative or causal relationship', such claims suggest that psychoactive drug (especially alcohol) use should be considered a major factor in the explanation of unsafe sexual practices.

Several other prominent researchers have contributed regularly to this debate with assertions that alcohol (and drug) use is a predictor of unsafe sexual behaviour. Among the most influential have been Stall and his associates in San Francisco. Most notably, Stall *et al.* (1986, p. 362) concluded from a particularly dated and methodologically suspect study of alcohol, amyl nitrite ('poppers') and marijuana use among gay men that: 'Depending on the specific drug, the men at high risk are from 2 to 3.5 times more likely to have used drugs during sexual activity than the men at no risk.'[2] Like Ostrow, Stall (1987) admits that his results should not be used to infer a causal connection between alcohol use and sexual behaviour, but this advice seems not to have been universally heeded. For example, the 'causative' link between drink and/or drugs and unsafe sex has now permeated much of the health promotion literature with admonitions to 'avoid' sex when drunk or high.

While most of these studies appear to show a statistical association between alcohol consumption and sexual practices, there still remains an unwarranted assumption that alcohol in some sense contributes to — or causes — people to engage in unsafe sexual practices. It is therefore important to note that the correlation is often made between gross alcohol intake in a given period (often a month) and the occurrence of 'risky' sex in the same period. What we are being asked to believe is that because an individual drank x units a week for a month and on one of those nights had 'risky' sex, that the former caused the latter. This stretches credibility to say the least.

It is particularly apposite to note that not only have some studies failed to replicate findings of a correlational relationship between unsafe sex and alcohol use (Leigh, 1990a, 1990b; see also Leigh, 1990c) but that in the only paper to distinguish between 'safe' and 'unsafe' sexual encounters and to examine the factors involved in those encounters, Gold *et al.* (1991, p. 14) say: 'The extent to which respondents had been under the influence of alcohol or drugs up to the start of sex, and the amount of alcohol, drugs or nitrites that they consumed during sex did not distinguish between the two types of encounter (safe/unsafe).' Leaving aside the question of what counts as 'risky' sex (see Chapter 10, this volume), it is possible to infer from the same correlation at least three causal structures. First, as is common, it may be inferred that alcohol consumption causes the risky sex. Second, and equally plausibly, the risky sex might cause the alcohol use ('My God, what have I done?'); or third, it might be a spurious effect: the individuals drink a lot and have risky sex for the same, underlying reason/s (cf. Jessor and Jessor, 1977).

One probable reason for preferring one causal inference rather than others is the vast literature on the disinhibiting effects of alcohol. The causal link is inferred because folk wisdom, stretching from the puritanical past, asserts the role of alcohol in breaking down the tenacity of the will. A plethora of studies (Solomon and Andrews, 1973; Room and Collins, 1983; Woods and Mansfield, 1983; O'Farrell *et al.*, 1983; Room, 1985; Reinarman and Leigh, 1987) suggests that alcohol has a disinhibiting effect on sexual behaviour. What does not appear so clearcut is whether alcohol makes people more likely to engage in what are now considered unsafe sexual practices. However, many articles make such a blind leap of faith as if evidence for disinhibitive effects is sufficient to 'explain' engagement in unsafe sexual practices. For example, Plant (1990, p. 295) justifiably asserts that 'the relevance to disinhibition to the AIDS epidemic is the *possibility* that people may be more likely to engage in "high risk" activities after drinking than they would otherwise be' [emphasis added],[3] but then proceeds as if such a possible effect was a certain or inevitable consequence of alcohol consumption.

We believe that this assumption is underpinned by the spurious notion that since people are on the whole well informed about HIV transmission, and are logical, rational and concerned for their own well-being, then there must be external factor/s that account for the enduring popularity of penetrative sex. Put simply, it is widely assumed that in the present situation engagement in penetrative and unprotected sexual intercourse — or 'casual sex', or commercial sex, depending on the particular axe you wish to grind — is both irresponsible and irrational. Hence people that continue to engage in such activities must suffer from some defect of the intellect (depression, suicidal tendencies, denial, etc.), or be under the influence of external factors (drugs, alcohol) that render them helpless to resist their baser instincts.

We favour a rather different perspective on the relationship between alcohol and unsafe sex. We believe that alcohol can function as an excuse for unsafe sex in that it can be presented as an abrogation of responsibility and a temporary interruption of rational control. This perspective derives from a different literature on the effects of alcohol from that which informs the orthodox account. For example, Crowe and George (1989, p. 382) described disinhibition effects as crucially revolving around a scapegoating or *self-excusing process*, in which 'feelings and actions are blamed on the liquor and so personally disavowed', or *social excusing*, that is, 'personal naughtiness will be misattributed by others to the alcohol and therefore excused by others because of it . . . [this] serves to evade attribution of responsibility to the self by society.'

Our data suggest that there is a range of disinhibitive effects which can be both social and sexual, and these may best be described as an 'activation of behaviours normally suppressed by various controlling influences' (Woods and Mansfield, 1983, p. 4). Our data also emphasize alcohol's role in enabling people to engage in behaviours they choose, rather than to obviate guilt or responsibility for personal actions which they, or others, find unacceptable.

Methods

Project SIGMA is a longitudinal study of a non-clinic-based cohort of homosexually active men.[4] Initiated in 1987 and currently funded until mid-1993, it has recruited over 1000 respondents by a variety of means including: (i) response to a postal questionnaire in the gay press; (ii) recruitment in gay pubs, clubs and social and political organizations; and (iii) through contacts of the above. These three sources each provided about one-third of respondents. Respondents lived in and around ten main sites across England and Wales: London, Cardiff, Newcastle, Teesside, Portsmouth, Leeds, Norwich, Birmingham, Liverpool and Bristol. No respondents were recruited from genito-urinary medicine clinics. Respondents have been interviewed at yearly intervals in 1988, 1989, 1990 and 1991. All four waves included detailed questions on alcohol use and sexual behaviour. Data presented here are from the first 392 respondents interviewed in 1990.

In this chapter we seek some understanding of the relationship/s between alcohol use and sexual behaviour. Distrustful of conventional and glib accounts of 'the' relationship between alcohol use and sexual behaviour, we have assumed that any relationship would not be simple, but complex and exceptionally difficult to measure.

The work of Project SIGMA differs from that which has gone before in two key respects: generally, it does not assume that the individual characteristics of persons are sufficient to explain the enduring popularity of unsafe sex, or that those persons that engage in unsafe sex have done so as a result of defects of character, intellect or weakness of resolve under the influence of alcohol (Davies and Weatherburn, 1991; Chapter, 10 this volume). Second, and more specifically, the research does not presume that there is strong interrelation between alcohol use and continued engagement in unsafe sex.

All 392 respondents interviewed in 1990 were asked a series of open-ended questions concerning their alcohol use and its effect on their sexual behaviour. The first question asked respondents was: '*Would you say alcohol plays a significant role in your sex life*? Those respondents who said 'yes', were probed in detail about its exact nature. Respondents were also asked whether alcohol had *ever* influenced them to engage in unsafe sexual behaviours. Rather than respondents being forced to choose any particular definition, they were allowed to define 'unsafe sexual behaviour'. Most respondents referred to *unprotected anal intercourse*, irrespective of partner type. Those respondents who had ever engaged in 'risky' sexual behaviour when they were intoxicated were asked how often this had happened, and the last time; how drunk would they say they were; what were the circumstances and the specific sexual behaviour involved; who with (casual or regular partner); whether the risk of HIV infection was considered; and whether orgasm was reached.

While this approach begins to give insight into the effects of alcohol on sexual behaviour, it is recognized that asking people retrospective questions about alcohol use may well be problematic, both because of social desirability phenomena and because alcohol itself impairs recall. While acknowledging these problems, we believe that the approach represents an improvement on more conventional methods, which involve researchers in making a leap of faith from quantitative estimates to possible scenarios or models, and in which correlational measures are used to impose an understanding of a situation over a respondent's own assessment of what happened.

Results

In the following discussion of our data we describe two aspects of the relationship between alcohol use and sexual behaviour. First, we consider the role that alcohol plays in the sexual lifestyle of men in the cohort, and find that it is complex and multifaceted. Second, we specifically consider the relationship between alcohol use and unsafe sex. While we rely upon reports of self-defined unsafe sex, the data suggest no reason to believe that the relationship would differ significantly if we used a more bio-medical definition of unsafe sex, such as unprotected anal intercourse.

Alcohol and Sexual Behaviour

Respondents were asked whether alcohol played a significant role in their sex lives. Of the 392 subjects questioned, 22.4 per cent (N = 88) stated that alcohol did so. The diversity and complexity of the interaction between alcohol and sexual behaviour can be seen in the differing roles and effects described by these men. Although, like Shakespeare, respondents distinguished many effects, five main roles are clearly discernible from the responses; and while some are interdependent, a vast majority of the respondents' explanations can be fitted to these roles without any difficulty. Only 25 per cent of responses related solely to one effect of alcohol use on the sexual behaviour of the men.

The first role revolves around *courage* and/or *relaxation of social inhibitions* and was mentioned by thirty-nine of the eighty-eight men (44 per cent) who ascribed a sexual role to their alcohol use, or an alcohol facet to their sexual lives.

A majority of these responses stressed alcohol's role of relaxing and aiding in the overcoming of social inhibitions:

> . . . makes me more relaxed and sociable.

> I can't talk to people unless I am drunk, I'd feel shy if I didn't drink I wouldn't have sex in [city X] without it. . . .

> I'm shy, it frees my inhibitions and makes me feel desirable. I don't get flustered. . . .

> Makes me less inhibited about talking with others. . . .

> Breaks down social inhibitions.

> Need a drink to relax me and make me uninhibited.

A similar but discernible social use revolves around alcohol's effects on confidence and courage:

> If I go cruising I wouldn't do it if I was sober, not confident enough. . . .

> Dutch courage, the ability to approach people.

> It helps me pluck up the courage to talk to someone.

It is worth noting that while none of these effects is necessarily incompatible with safer sexual practices, alcohol is used to facilitate sexual contacts. One could argue that if alcohol is used to overcome crises of confidence and instill courage, it may serve to empower and enable people who choose to engage in safer sexual practices but find it difficult to negotiate such encounters. For example, one man stressed that he was 'more assertive and less shy when drunk.'

The second, complementary and sometimes indiscernible role revolves around the *relaxation of sexual inhibitions* as mentioned by seven (8 per cent) of the eighty-eight men who ascribed a sexual role to their alcohol use. While this role may be inferred from some of the quotes in the 'social inhibitions' section, we only counted those quotes that have explicit sexual connotations.

> It has quite a large role in that it lowers my inhibitions: I do more and am more adventurous.

> . . . makes my partner less inhibited: the chances of getting anything out of him are rare unless he's had a few.

> I do not use drink for my own release but as a way of releasing my partner's inhibitions . . . puts him in the mood.

I like to have sex if I've had a drink. Less discriminate about who I do it with. Not that important who with as long as they do the chasing.

As a general disinhibitor. I'm more likely to have sex with someone if I've been drinking, but not necessarily.

More likely to indulge in casual sex after a drink, but not really a great role. Marginally disinhibiting.

Makes me more receptive to receptive anal intercourse, it relaxes me. . . .

There seems to be a disinhibition effect for at least half the men that ascribe a sexual role to alcohol use. That is, some respondents drink in order to muster the confidence or courage to 'pick up' or be 'picked up', or to be more sexually adventurous. Either way, the use of alcohol seems to be deliberate and premeditated.

The third role revolves around effects on *sexual performance*. Forty-one of the eighty-eight men (47 per cent) mentioned this. Of these, 50 per cent described a negative effect on sexual performance, 21 per cent a positive effect and 29 per cent an equivocal effect. Comments identifying negative effects on performance included:

. . . sex is better without alcohol: it is difficult to obtain an erection and it takes longer to reach orgasm.

. . . I like drinking but it makes my sex worse.

... alcohol tires me out: I get into something then my head spins and I don't know what I'm doing. It hinders me, makes me tired so I can't be bothered to perform.

. . . nothing works if I'm pissed.

It inhibits performance: I can still do it but don't enjoy it. It doesn't enhance it.

. . . drink makes me less sexually arousable.

Those highlighting positive effects on performance suggested:

Enhances performance . . .

. . . prolongs the sex.

I'm better when I've had a few drinks.

Whereas mixed effects on performance suggested:

Sex is good at the end of a good night out but the effect varies: too much and too little alters my performance.

. . . not as potent but I can last longer.

Clearly alcohol does not have a unitary effect on sexual performance: in differing amounts it has differing effects on different people; while half the men interviewed report the expected negative effect on arousal, erection, ejaculation and/or lethargy, the other half report generally positive or negligible effects.

Alcohol's effects on sexual performance are interlinked with the fourth role which revolves around its effects on *sexual desire*. Thirteen of the eighty-eight men (15 per cent) mentioned this.

Being quite tipsy increases the desire. . . .

Makes me horny.

Get really randy when I drink and want to bed anything in sight. . . .

Improves my randiness and enthusiasm. . . .

Urge to fuck is greater when drunk but I've managed to resist so far.

Regular partner doesn't drink but I use it as an aid to sex. It can add a new dimension to sex.

A very minor role, want more [sex] with my regular partner at home, when I've had a drink or two.

. . . in the right amount, it would make me want sex . . .

Often with regular partner I have a drink before; it puts me on a high straight away and makes me feel sensual but it isn't an integral part of sex, and it isn't necessary. . . .

. . . increases libido.

Although alcohol may or may not 'take away the performance', at least among some people, it certainly provokes the desire.

The fifth role revolves around the use of alcohol in the *social scene*. Twenty of the eighty-eight men (23 per cent) mentioned this.

The gay scene is drink orientated as only places to meet are bars and clubs. . . .

Linked with social life. . . .

Don't use alcohol to have sex but most cruising is in bars.

I meet people in pubs, drink helps me to meet people.

Meet at pubs and clubs. It is not a requirement to meet but I use bars and clubs to pick up.

Only in forging contacts in pubs and clubs.

Many times when I have sex with others I have been drinking because in a bar or pub to pick them up. . . .

Drinking is merely part of the social background. . . .

Alcohol and sexual behaviour may be linked merely because in those places where initial sexual contacts are commonly forged — pubs, clubs, parties — alcohol use is an integral part of the social milieu. In these circumstances the effects of alcohol consumption are difficult to judge precisely, but given the prevalence of its use as a social disinhibitor, it would be misleading to suggest that it caused people to have sex.

Only six of the eighty-eight men (7 per cent) specifically mentioned the effect/non-effect of alcohol on their actual sexual behaviour, and of these only one mentioned that alcohol '*makes them*' have sex they would not have had otherwise: '. . . Don't worry about safe sex so much when drunk.' The other five men described effects that are far more difficult to classify.

Makes sex more enjoyable and changes my sexual behaviour.

Though it helps me to chat to people, when I take people home it does not change my sexual behaviour with them.

. . . it doesn't affect the sex I have with people.

It has made me do things I wouldn't normally do.

Makes me more passive: with it I like being fucked but always use condoms.

Alcohol Use and 'Risky' Sex

In the last section it was suggested that the relationship between alcohol use and sex is complex. Alcohol not only has different effects on different people, it also has different effects on the same people at different times. It therefore seems premature for researchers to talk of a relationship between unsafe sex and alcohol before the relationship between sex and alcohol is more clearly appreciated.

It is incontrovertible that unsafe sex does happen when at least one of the participants has been drinking. Thirty-seven per cent (N = 145) of this sample stated that they had *ever* engaged in 'risky' sexual behaviour when they were not completely sober. However, among those that had, in their own terms, behaved riskily there was considerable variation in the number of times they had done so, in what sex had taken place and in the context/s within which it had occurred.

Type of Sex. Almost two-thirds (64 per cent) of these sexual encounters (from just eighty-eight (22 per cent) of the men in the cohort) involved anal intercourse, and about a fifth (18 per cent) involved fellatio to orgasm. Of those men who had

engaged in anal intercourse when intoxicated, only 14 per cent had used a condom, even though these acts culminated in orgasm on a majority (86 per cent) of
occasions. This represents a very high incidence of anal intercourse compared to
the cohort as a whole (Davies *et al.*, 1990) and a very low figure for condom use
(Weatherburn *et al.*, 1991). Nevertheless, given that respondents were asked to
recall an unsafe encounter, it is perhaps noteworthy that only two-thirds involved
anal intercourse. There is some, admittedly inconclusive, evidence from this data
that when 'unsafe' sex happens while intoxicated, men move one step down what
could be termed the sex safety scale. That is, those who would not normally let
someone come in their mouth would do so, but would not get fucked, say.
Similarly, someone who would normally use a condom might not do so. While
this may be considered an emergent hypothesis at best, it is worthy of future
consideration.

Context. The diverse and multifaceted association/s between alcohol use and sexual
behaviour are probably better illustrated by a selection of the descriptions of these
'unsafe' encounters. Respondents who reported an 'unsafe' encounter were asked
to describe the circumstances including how inebriated they felt, whether they
considered or discussed the risk of HIV infection, and the type of partner the
encounter occurred with. Less than half of the respondents recounted encounters
where they were incapable of negotiating safer sex — even if they had wished to
— or when they subsequently regretted having had unsafe sex.

> Falling down drunk in [cruising area] I had receptive anal intercourse
> with a regular partner and didn't care about the risks.

> In June 1987 — very drunk, too drunk to think clearly but have regretted
> it since. Had receptive anal intercourse with a casual partner who was
> foreign.

On the other hand, a majority recounted an unsafe encounter in which they
had quite deliberately and consciously decided to engage in the sexual activity
described.

> Though I was fairly drunk wasn't staggering. We both claimed to be
> negative [HIV antibody status] and took each other's word for it and had
> anal intercourse without a condom.

> Quite pissed but not too drunk to think clearly and I would have done
> it if I was sober. Met a new partner in a club and had anal intercourse
> without orgasm and with a condom.

> I was very drunk. I did say that I didn't really want to and he said he
> didn't really like using condoms so I said what the hell.

> Not out of my head but quite drunk and relaxed. I was able to think
> about the risk. It was with casual partners, about three or four times a
> couple of years ago. Anal intercourse without condoms, but without
> coming inside each other.

I was reasonably drunk, but not so drunk that I didn't know what was happening. A couple of months ago with my regular partner, at his place, we both got very drunk and had anal intercourse without a condom. I was slightly worried afterwards. Drink certainly influenced it.

Among all the men who had engaged in unsafe sex when under the influence of alcohol, attitudes to safer sex varied considerably. While some said that the encounter had been the result of a grave error of judgment on their part, others were quite blase about the risks they had taken and did not feel that their sexual behaviour — or alcohol use — were problematic. Clearly, then, there are substantial individual differences that need to be taken into account when examining both why and under what circumstances adherence to safer sex guidelines is suspended or abandoned.

Of those men that considered the HIV-related risks, and under the circumstances decided to have sex, it could be argued that alcohol has a clear social and/or sexual disinhibition effect. However, it does not follow that alcohol 'caused' these men to have unsafe sex; indeed, it may have enabled them to engage in sexual activities that they had consciously and rationally decided that they wished to engage in. As can be seen from the data above, some men use alcohol in a premeditated way to facilitate sexual contact/s or to enable them to engage in activities that would otherwise be problematic.

However, some respondents articulated incidents when they were too drunk to think clearly, and/or so drunk that they engaged in sexual activities which they subsequently regretted. We would argue that for these men alcohol still cannot be said to have 'caused' them to engage in unsafe sex; but there appears to be some relationship between unsafe sex and alcohol consumption, and alcohol perhaps plays a very different role in their social and sexual lives. In the sense that these men may not have made a conscious choice to engage in unsafe sex — though not necessarily irrational — they might benefit from health promotion interventions that include, though not necessarily overemphasize, the possible role of psychoactive drugs in sexual activity.

Conclusions

The relationship between alcohol consumption and sexual behaviour is complex, variable and far from fully understood. The effects of alcohol on sexual desire, inhibitions and performance vary greatly across individuals. They also depend crucially on the context of the sexual encounter and the other party involved in the sexual negotiation: after all, unsafe sex cannot be managed alone. As one particularly perceptive respondent pointed out: 'It all depends what I want to do, who I'm with, where I am. . . .' However, there is undoubtedly some relationship, at least for some pairs in some circumstances; and health educators, in particular, could benefit from understanding it more clearly. However, in order to make a fair and objective assessment of this relationship, we need to suspend previous judgments, especially those based on puritanical preconceptions and popular myth.

One of the most notable aspects of the data presented is that they are not all about alcohol's effects on the reporter, nor are they all regarding 'casual' sex or 'casual' sexual partners. In the SIGMA data men commonly report the uses and effects of alcohol on their partners and/or their sexual (and social) interaction with their partners. These aspects of the connection between alcohol use and sexual behaviour have rarely been considered, perhaps because it is so commonly assumed that the problem is the association between alcohol use and engagement in casual sex. Thus it is usually assumed that people who would not normally have unsafe sex, drink and then have unsafe sex 'against their better judgment'. The fact that they have consumed alcohol not only allows them and others to 'excuse' their behaviour, but also it provides health educators with a focus for intervention that, we argue, may not be particularly useful. Thus although alcohol use may be problematic for some men who have sex with men, its connection with sexual behaviour is complex and poorly understood, and its use as an explanation for engagement in 'unsafe' sexual practices may be misleading and dangerous.

Even if it were the case that alcohol use and engagement in unsafe sex were consistently correlated, no one has considered the benefits of alcohol use and its facilitative effects, even though one might assume that, given its enduring popularity, people feel it is worth the financial and health-related costs. In short, scientists have simplified the relationship between alcohol use and sexual behaviour and evacuated the rational from the decision-making process. What we are doing is to rehumanize the argument which in the most common version is naïvely empirical and of dubious utility for HIV/AIDS health promotion.

Notes

1 At present Project SIGMA is Paul Broderick, Tony Coxon, Peter Davies, Ford Hickson, Andrew Hunt, Tom McManus, Michael Stephens and Peter Weatherburn.
2 The study is dated because the HIV risks assigned to acts are, in retrospect, wrong. More importantly, it is flawed because the risk index created uses arbitrary weighting criteria to describe 'no', 'medium' and 'high' risk behaviours.
3 See also Robertson and Plant (1988); Plant *et al.* (1990); Bagnall *et al.* (1990).
4 *Socio-sexual Investigations of Gay Men and AIDS.*

References

BAGNALL, G., PLANT, M.A. and WARWICK, W. (1990) 'Alcohol, Drugs and AIDS-related Risks: Results from a Prospective Study', *AIDS Care*, 2, pp. 309–17.
CROWE, L.C. and GEORGE, W.H. (1989) 'Alcohol and Human Sexuality: Review and Integration', *Psychological Bulletin*, 105, 3, pp. 374–86.
DAVIES, P.W. and WEATHERBURN, P. (1991) 'Towards a General Model of Sexual Negotiation', in P. AGGLETON, P. DAVIES and G. HART (Eds), *AIDS: Responses, Policy and Care*, Lewes, Falmer Press.
DAVIES, P.M., HUNT, A.J., MACOURT, M. and WEATHERBURN P. (1990) 'A Longitudinal Study of the Sexual Behaviour of Homosexual Males under the Impact of AIDS: A Final Report Submitted to the Department of Health', London, Project SIGMA.
GOLDBECK, A.L. and MOLGAARD, C.A. (1990) 'Methodological Issues Concerning the

Sensitive Query in AIDS/Alcohol Research: Sample Size Estimates for Randomized Response Procedures', in D. SEMINARA, R.R. WATSON and A. PAWLOWSKI (Eds), *Alcohol, Immunomodulation, and AIDS*, New York, Allan Liss, pp. 35–46.

GOLD, R.S., SKINNER, M.S., GRANT, P.J. and PLUMMER, D.C. (1991) 'Situational Factors and Thought Processes Associated with Unprotected Intercourse in Gay Men', *Psychology and Health*, 5 (in press).

HINGSON, R., STRUNIN, L., BERLIN, B. and HEEREN, T. (1990) 'Beliefs about AIDS, Use of Alcohol, Drugs and Unprotected Sex among Massachusetts Adolescents', *American Journal of Public Health*, 80, pp. 295–9.

JESSOR, R. and JESSOR, S.L. (1977) *Problem Behaviour Psychosocial Development: A Longitudinal Study of Youth*, New York, Academic Press.

LEIGH, B.C. (1990a) 'The Relationships of Substance Use during Sex to High-risk Sexual Behaviour', *Journal of Sex Research*, 27, pp. 199–213.

LEIGH, B.C. (1990b) 'The Relationship of Sex-related Alcohol Expectancies to Alcohol Consumption and Sexual Behaviour', *British Journal of Addiction*, 85, pp. 919–28.

LEIGH, B.C. (1990c) 'Alcohol and Unsafe Sex: An Overview of Research and Theory', in D. SEMINARA, R.R. WATSON and A. PAWLOWSKI (Eds), *Alcohol, Immunomodulation, and AIDS*, New York, Alan R. Liss.

O'FARRELL, J.J., WEYLAND, C.A. and LOGAN, D. (1983) *Alcohol and Sexuality: An Annotated Bibliography on Alcohol Use, Alcoholism and Human Sexual Behaviour*, Phoenix, Ariz., Oryx Press.

OSTROW, D.G. (1986) 'Barriers to the Recognition of Links between Drug and Alcohol Abuse and AIDS', in *Acquired Immune Deficiency Syndrome and Chemical Dependency*, DHHS Pub. No. ADM 87–1513, Washington, D.C., US Government Printing Office.

PLANT, M.A. (1990) 'Alcohol, Sex and AIDS', *Alcohol and Alcoholism*, 25, pp. 293–301.

PLANT, M.L., PLANT, M.A. and MORGAN THOMAS, R. (1990) 'Alcohol, AIDS Risks and Commercial Sex: Some Preliminary Results from a Scottish Study', *Drug and Alcohol Dependence*, 25, pp. 51–5.

REINARMAN, C. and LEIGH, B.C. (1987) 'Culture, Cognition, and Disinhibition: Notes on Sexuality and Alcohol in the Age of AIDS', *Contemporary Drug Problems*, 14, pp. 435–60.

ROBERTSON, J.A. and PLANT, M.A. (1988) 'Alcohol, Sex and Risks of HIV Infection', *Drug and Alcohol Dependence*, 22, pp. 75–8.

ROOM, R. (1985) 'AIDS and Alcohol: Epidemiological and Behavioural Aspects', Paper prepared for NIAAA consultation on AIDS and Alcohol, 4–5 November, Berkeley, California.

ROOM, R. and COLLINS, G. (Eds) (1983) 'Introduction', in *Alcohol and Disinhibition: Nature and Meaning of the Link*, NIAAA Research Monograph 12, Washington, D.C., NIAAA.

SOLOMON, D. and ANDREWS, G. (1973) *Drugs and Sexuality*, Herts, Panther.

STALL, R. (1987) 'The Prevention of HIV Infection Associated with Drug and Alcohol Use during Sexual Activity', in L. Seigel (Ed.), *AIDS and Substance Abuse*, New York, Harrington Park Press.

STALL, R., McKUSICK, L., WILEY, J., COATES, T. and OSTROW, D. (1986) 'Alcohol and Drug Use during Sexual Activity and Compliance with Safe Sex Guidelines for AIDS: The AIDS Behavioural Research Project', *Health Education Quarterly*, 13, pp. 359–71.

VALDISSERRI, R.O., LYTER, D., LEVITON, L.C., et al. (1988) 'Variables Influencing Condom Use in a Cohort of Gay and Bisexual Men', *American Journal of Public Health*, 78, pp. 801–5.

WEATHERBURN, P., HUNT, A.J., DAVIES, P.M., COXON, A.P.M. and McMANUS, T.J.

(1991) 'Condom Use in a Large Cohort of Homosexually Active Males', *AIDS Care*, 3, 1, pp. 31–41.

WOODS, S.C. and MANSFIELD, J.G. (1983) 'Ethanol and Disinhibition: Psychological and Behavioural Links', in R. ROOM and G. COLLINS (Eds), *Alcohol and Disinhibition: Nature and Meaning of the Link*, NIAAA Research Monograph 12, Washington, D.C., NIAAA.

10   On Relapse: Recidivism or Rational Response?

Peter Davies and Project SIGMA[1]

A number of behavioural studies tracking the response of gay and bisexual men to AIDS have commented on an increase over the last one to three years in the percentage of men reporting anal intercourse and, in particular, a number of men fucking in the late 1980s, who in the mid-1980s were not doing so. Most researchers (e.g., Stall *et al.*, 1990 Sherr and Strong, 1990; Adib *et al.*, 1991) have taken these data to indicate that gay and bisexual men are 'relapsing' to unsafe sex.[2] This notion of relapse threatens to inform the next generation of health education initiatives for gay and bisexual men, yet it remains a beguiling but imprecise idea that is conceptually untenable, empirically dubious and politically naïve.

The Concept

The term 'relapse' canonically refers to the reappearance of the signs or symptoms of a disease after a period of absence or remission. It was taken up by scientists in the 1960s to refer to people who began to drink or use drugs after a period of abstinence. This use arose out of the redefinition of alcoholism and drug addiction (sic) as somatic disease states (see Jellinek, 1960) rather than moral or personality effects. The disease could be symptomatic (i.e., the patient was drinking) or asymptomatic (s/he was not doing so). The term gradually replaced the earlier term 'recidivism', which indicated a willed, indeed wilful return to the former behaviour. Behind the term 'relapse' in this context is the idea that a basic drive — the need for drink/drugs — has triumphed over the 'rational' decision to abstain and so signifies a loss of control by the mind over the body.

The term 'relapse' has now been applied to unsafe/risky sex. It is useful to spell out what use of the term entails. It says that gay and bisexual men are unable to maintain the patterns of safer sexual behaviour for which they have been widely praised. They are, the term asserts, falling victim again to their urges, unable to resist a damned good fuck in the interests of their individual safety and the greater good. As Gary Dowsett comments elsewhere in this volume (see Chapter 1), 'relapse' is not a term that would be used of the sexual behaviour of heterosexual men or women and is indicative of a subtle homophobia. It is, therefore, deeply distressing to see gay academics and researchers promulgating the use of the term.

Presumably, those who talk about 'relapse' into unsafe sex do not really see sex as a disease, but what do they mean? We suggest that relapse emerges from two pervasive but fundamentally misdirected patterns of thought which we will term the individualist and the romantic fallacies.

The Individualist Fallacy

Elsewhere (Davies and Weatherburn, 1991) we have commented at length on the provenance, predominance and pervasiveness of individual explanations of sexual behaviour in general and unsafe behaviour in particular. Unsafe sexual behaviour is caused, we are asked to believe, by deficiencies of the individual, by his lack of knowledge (although it seems hypocritical to condemn our respondent for not knowing what unsafe sex is, when the 'experts' themselves are hardly clearer); by inappropriate or incorrect beliefs or attitudes, as suggested by the Health Belief Model (Rosenstock, 1974; Fitzpatrick, Boulton and Hart, 1989) an the AIDS Risk Reduction Model (Catania *et al.*, 1990) or the theory of planned behaviour (Ajzen and Madden, 1986); by lack of self-control of self-efficacy, especially under the influence of alcohol or drugs; or by an inability to put intentions into practice. The upshot of this focus on individual factors, motivations and abilities, buttressed by impressive statistical apparatus, is that unsafe sex is something that we do by ourselves. While it is not only possible but very common to have sex alone, the notion of having unsafe sex by oneself is simply bizarre.

This concentration on the individual is fundamentally misguided. Sex is, after language, the most *inter*personal of human activities. It is, in its myriad diversities, an exchange of pleasure, a negotiation of desire, a sharing of self and body. The progress of a sexual session is a physical conversation, within which fucking plays an important role, with different meaning and connotation in different circumstances. Men fuck as a result of an ongoing, explicit or implicit negotiation between (at least) two individuals.

It is true that the paradigm models of risk reduction usually incorporate some measure of communication skill, but two problems render this inclusion spurious and ultimately unhelpful. First, the measures explicitly or implicitly (implicit, often in the illustrative material which accompanies the analysis) assume that the negotiation of safer sex is verbal. It seems to be assumed that the conversation — 'Shall we use a condom, then?' 'Yeh, why not' — is the limit of 'negotiation'. In the data emerging from Project SIGMA (see below) two-thirds of those who had had what they regarded as unsafe sex said that they had not talked about the sort of sex they were going to have, yet they had engaged in a non-verbal, physical negotiation. Each sexual session is the result of a negotiation which continues from before the physical connection is made to the post-coital cigarette.

Second, while an individual can be thought to have better or worse communication skills, it is surely inappropriate to suppose that he will always be able equally to put them into practice. Within a given relationship an individual will find himself sometimes in control of the situation, at other times under the control of his partner. It is important to recognize that sexual negotiation, while universal, is not necessarily between *equals*. Age differences, racial differences, disparities in social or economic status, sexual attractiveness, sexual role, etc. all create sexual situations in which one individual becomes more able to dictate the course of events than does the other, though these abilities are not fixed, even between two individuals.

The relapse theory commits the individualistic fallacy in looking for the reasons for renewed fucking in the deficiencies of individuals: low self-esteem, self-efficacy, poor community integration, the tendency to drink or use drugs. We want to be clear that we believe it far more fruitful to seek the *cause* of particular sexual behaviour in the interaction between individuals, not their psychological mal-functioning.

The Romantic Fallacy

Not only do the dominant models of relapse in particular and unsafe sex in general concentrate on the individual to an unwarranted extent; they also perpetuate the notion that sex is 'natural', overwhelming and supremely irrational or, at best, non-rational. It is worth examining some of the strands of this belief in the hope that scrutiny will at least make explicit some of the assumptions which it involves.

First, two millenia of Christian thought have urged the subservience of the body to the will. The origins of this belief in the first three centuries of the common era derive from a particular model of the relationship between the body and the spirit, but its ossification over centuries of Christian thought has led to the belief becoming deeply ingrained in the Western mind that the body's demands — lust, thirst, pleasure, etc. — are undesirable, indeed evil and subhuman drives to be controlled by the will.

The second strand is the romantic tradition, dating, according to preference, from the twelfth or the nineteenth century, with its characterization of love as an overwhelming passion over which one has no control (hence falling in love; love will find a way) and which cannot be denied (Lancelot is literally driven mad by his unrequited love for Guinevere). The romantic tradition exalts the paradox of the proximity of the lowest of base instincts and the 'highest of human emotions'.

Unsafe sexual behaviour, especially fucking without a condom, is seen in the dominant paradigm as a basic (irrational) drive which the (rational) will is constantly striving to control. Prieur's (1990) important work on the meaning of fucking to gay men emphasizes the naturalness of the experience. Safer sex is seen as a necessary but unpleasant course of action which is dictated by prudence rather than desire (Pollak, 1988). We may distinguish two corollaries of this attitude which are of particular moment.

First, it is assumed that safer sex is *the* rational choice. No one could possibly *choose* to have unsafe sex or make a conscious and reasoned decision to fuck. This fallacy rests on a fundamental misunderstanding of the term 'rational', which we shall take up below. Second, it leads to a conception of safer sex as a strategy of control, both at the individual level and, by extension, at the social, normative level. In particular, monogamy features as a preferred response to AIDS, and a distressing number of recent papers and contributions bury their moral agenda in their criteria of 'unsafe sex'. Third, the goal of the paradigm model seems to be the eradication of fucking among gay men. Quite apart from the homophobia which this attitude displays, it is an impractical and undesirable goal, for reasons which we now examine.

Taken together, the romantic and the individual fallacies generate two paradigms of relapse. The first is the more popular and underpins much of the explanatory gloss with which the advocates of 'relapse' accompany their figures. This is the 'heat of the moment' scenario. A man, often drunk or high, finds himself (the lack of agency is indicative) in a 'hot' encounter and fucks or is fucked. This scenario, which Jane Mezzone (personal communication) has referred to as the 3-D syndrome (it was dark, I was drunk and I didn't know what I was doing), is one which no doubt occurs, but which, as we shall argue from a consideration of Project SIGMA's data, is very infrequent. The second stereotype is the 'habitual' relapser, who denies or fatalistically accepts the possibility of infection and fucks with whomsoever he can.

However, these explanations at best only tell half the story. Since the concept of relapse focuses on a group of men who 'cannot say no' to fucking, it presumes, but ignores, another group who ask them to say 'yes' to fucking. Where and who are they? Rather than think in terms of these groups of men, one present and pilloried in the literature, the other unaccountably invisible, it is more fruitful to seek the particular *circumstances* which are conducive to unsafe sex.

Rationality

The notion of rationality lies at the heart of the debate about safer sexual practice in particular and behaviour which minimizes the risk of HIV transmission in general. Yet the concept is often used in a contradictory and confusing manner, which muddies the debate and is unhelpful in the urgent task of understanding, establishing and reinforcing safer sexual behaviour.

Perhaps the most insidious and pervasive misuse of the term 'rational' is that which confuses the process of decision-making with the decision itself. When used correctly, the term refers to the process, not the outcome. Thus a decision is rational if it is made after a consideration of the available evidence in the light of the circumstances pertaining at the time. By contrast, an irrational decision is one which ignores, dismisses or otherwise deems irrelevant available information.

The eventual decision — which we will take, for the sake of exemplar and without loss of generality, to be a decision to fuck — may, in addition, be right or wrong according to epidemiological or other criteria, but the rationality of the decision process is independent of the rightness of the outcome. Thus an individual can (i) rationally come to the right decision, (ii) irrationally come to the right decision; (iii) rationally come to the wrong decision; (iv) irrationally come to the wrong decision. The criteria on which we decide whether a decision is right or wrong and the criteria by which we decide if a process is rational or irrational are distinct.

Rationality and Heuristic

Even among those writers who correctly use 'rational' to refer to the process of decision-making there is a further tendency to use an unrealistically complex version of the decision-making process. They regard individuals as making rational decisions on the basis of detailed epidemiological data and sophisticated models of contagion and infection which are simply outside the scope of the ordinary person in the street or bedroom.

In this version the decision process is often represented as a choice, either to fuck or not to do so. Each choice carries with it a probability of becoming infected with HIV (if currently uninfected) or of passing it on (if currently infected). Thus there are four possible outcomes: (i) fucking and passing the virus; (ii) fucking and not passing the virus; (iii) not fucking and passing the virus; and (iv) not fucking and not passing the virus. Each of the four outcomes has a unique utility to the individual which is a function of three values: the utility of infection; the utility of the fuck; and the probability of infection. The rational man or woman will choose the outcome with the greatest terminal utility.

It is often unclear whether the model is being used descriptively — a representation of what actually happens — or prescriptively — a description of the truly rational response. As a descriptive method, it fails for a number of reasons, particularly when applied to sexual behaviour. First, the decision to fuck is not made once and for all at some point in the preamble — or, if you are energetic, the run-up — to sex; nor indeed during the 'foreplay'. The decision to fuck is continuously made throughout the session, and the intention can and does change from second to second during that time. Second, the decision or decisions to fuck are not made by individuals, they are made by (at least) two people who are engaged in a complex social negotiation, which we understand poorly. Third, and most crucially, the rational decision-making model fails as a description of the decision-making process because individuals do not have perfect knowledge, they work with subjective probabilities and assess the various elements of the model in different and sometimes idiosyncratic ways.

A common assumption of the researchers using the rational model is that the utility of infection — or, more accurately, its disutility — is so overwhelming that the transient pleasure of a mere fuck cannot, rationally, ever outweigh the potential devastation of infection. This is a bloodless and arrogant view, yet it underpins the agenda which sees the eradication of HIV transmission as following from the eradication of fucking among gay men. Where the choice is starkest, say among street children, it is surely an entirely rational decision to be fucked if the alternative is to starve. Having said that, the choice between the possibility of a slow death in a number of years and the certainty of death now is one which all of us should be ashamed to impose on anyone. To add to that the arrogance of dismissing the validity of choice is inexcusable.

Third, the failure of the model as a descriptive tool lies in its elision of the fact that individuals make choices, not on the basis of accurate information — your average man in the cottage does not anxiously peruse the *British Medical Journal* to assess the prevalence of HIV infection in his locality — but on the basis of heuristic rules. Thus the common decision in the early years of the epidemic in Britain not to fuck with Americans was a relatively good heuristic device which recognized the difference in prevalence between the two countries. On the other hand, cues such as the physical appearance of an individual or his perceived lifestyle are relatively poor heuristic devices and are rightly discouraged by some health promotion interventions.

Recidivism

As we have noted above, the term 'relapse' entered behavioural science as the attempt was made to cast alcoholism and drug addiction as diseases. In that process the term 'recidivism' fell out of use. Usually used to signify apostasy or the renunciation of recantation — a return to a formerly rejected heresy — it entails a conscious decision to return to old ways. While usually used pejoratively to signify wilful disrespect for socially sanctioned behaviour or belief, recidivism can also indicate the assertion of individual principle over social pressure to conform. If we really need a term to describe what is happening at the moment, then recidivism, with its overtones of conscious moral choice, is surely to be preferred.

To see relapse as a momentary lapse of concentration or of the will absolves both the man involved and the social scientist on the sidelines of the need to think about safer sex not as an isolated instance of wild abandon — over which he has no control — but as an act or acts that emerge from decisions taken, perhaps in the heat of the moment, and for the consequences of which he must take responsibility. Safer sex is therefore a long-term strategy of maximization of pleasure and prudence.

Empirical Evidence

For the above reasons we believe the notion of 'relapse' in relation to what is happening among gay men to be theoretically unsound.[3] From our own data we also believe it to be empirically dubious. Descriptions of the SIGMA cohort may be found elsewhere (Davies *et al.*, 1990; Chapter 9, this volume). The data used in this paper refer to 699 men interviewed in 1988 and 1989. The average time between interviews was ten months. Between 1988 and 1990 we find a small net increase in the proportion of men who report fucking (either insertive or receptive or both) in the month before interview from 41 per cent (289/699) to 43 per cent (301/699).

It is a part of the dominant relapse paradigm that there is a small proportion of hard to reach or recalcitrant gay and bisexual men who continue to fuck. The increase in the proportion of men fucking is then seen as an increase in the size of this small group and a defeat for health promotion initiatives. This interpretation is simply not borne out by the data. The proportion of men fucking in both years is only 14 per cent (96/699), and 29 per cent (205/699) of the men in the study have not fucked in the two years. Some men are giving it up and others are taking it up. Perhaps most importantly, it is not possible to distinguish statistically between the men who have begun to fuck in terms of self-efficacy ($F = 1.65$; $p = .26$), perceived social norms ($F = .48$; $p = .70$), sex communication skills ($F = 2.02$; $p = .11$), enjoyment of anal intercourse ($F = .11$; $p = .95$) or perceived riskiness of anal intercourse ($F = 1.13$; $p = .34$).

The importance of this result cannot be overstressed. If relapse is to have any meaning, then we should be able to find some characteristics of the individuals who have relapsed which are at least associated with, perhaps even play a causative role in, explaining the re-emergence of unsafe behaviour. This is not so in this cohort.

On the other hand, if one uses log-linear analysis of the proportions fucking in wave 1 and 2, 93 per cent of the increase can be accounted for by increases in regular sexual relationships. This result needs also to be assessed. It is not the case that a regular relationship is a risk factor, nor, indeed, that love is a risk factor. What this indicates is, in broad terms, that understanding the re-emergence of unsafe sex requires a consideration of interpersonal, not individual factors and that safer sex is not only an avoidance of some and a preference for other sexual practices, but a patterning of sexual relationships in a long- or at least medium-term strategy.

We also record that while 34 per cent fucked or were fucked in 1988, only 1.2 per cent were fucked without a condom by a non-regular partner. Taken together, we conclude from this patterning that the increase in fucking is not a result of psychological malfunction but of conscious choice in real circumstances. Individuals are not making a once and for all assessment of their risk of contracting or passing on HIV. Nor do they make a once and for all assessment of the possibility of transmitting the virus with this or that partner. Rather, the assessment of personal risk and susceptibility is made dynamically, varying from minute to minute before and after, and arguably from second to second within the sexual encounter.

In our analysis of risk perception and the evaluation of susceptibility, we want to steer a middle course between those who see the process as a supremely rational one, where the individual makes a decision simply on the basis of the probability of infection, the disutility of infection and the utility of the fuck to come, and those who see the process as a non-rational, intuitive one where the body rules the mind. We believe that the assessment of risk is made on heuristic grounds and some of those grounds are more robust than others. Some writers have argued that certain cues are inappropriate — looks, attitude, willingness to fuck, etc., but these are exactly the sort of cues that people do use and which need to be addressed. The relapse model diverts attention from this process in a way that is unhelpful and unscientific. It provides the individual with a ready-made excuse — the 3-D syndrome — for unsafe behaviour, which fails to address the real reasons for a regretted episode.

Three points need to be made. First, there is no doubt that the 3-D syndrome does happen. There will always be a few occasions when we fuck against our better judgment. We propose that it is neither the only nor the most important explanation for what we see in terms of increases in the rate of unsafe sex. Note also the formulation of the sentence. It is not the case that there are a few individuals who are prone to or habitually relapse — or if there are, they are very rare — but that this is a situation in which all of us can, and many of us will, find ourselves.

Second, the decision to fuck with a regular partner is not necessarily a 'safe' choice. The long latency period of the virus and eternal relativity of trust make the decision one which is made on probabilistic rather than absolute information. But the relapse model absolves both those who fuck and researchers from acknowledging gay men's — our — right to fuck. One eminent researcher, in a recent conversation, was unable to say what she regarded as a safe or acceptable level of fucking in the homosexual population. This indicates to my suspicious mind at least that the only safe strategy is to eliminate fucking as a practice among gay men. Quite apart from the blatant homophobia of this goal, it is simply unrealistic, yet it lies at the heart of the correlational research paradigm that fills the journals and dominates the conferences.

Third, in asserting the right of gay men to fuck, we do not naïvely believe that the choice to fuck is made freely by all men in all situations. We may be forced to fuck, we may force others to fuck, but we believe that an explanation of sexual behaviour in general and fucking in particular is to be found in the dynamics of the interaction, not in the psychology of individuals.

Practical and Political

We have already indicated that one result of the relapse model is to absolve individuals and researchers from confronting the reality of the decision to fuck, when that decision had led to an incident that is later regretted. In this way the responsibility for that decision can also be evaded. Moreover, by providing a ready-made rationale which emphasizes the irrational and the animal nature, it impedes rather than encourages the clarification of motive and cause which is the end of reflection.

One practical effect of the relapse model is to repathologize gay men. By emphasizing the 'failure to maintain' safer sex, this paradigm highlights deficiencies in the individual on which tried and tested interventions can be focused. No doubt somebody, somewhere is even now implementing twelve-step programmes to help men who cannot help fucking. Such interventions are popular, since they rely on existing models of individual change. There is nothing intrinsically wrong with a programme which elucidates and makes explicit the decision processes which lead to unwanted fucking, but they are to be regarded in the present circumstances as unhelpful for at least two reasons. First, to be admitted to such a programme a man has to label himself as deficient. This is unhelpful to that individual and absolves those who do not, or will not, see themselves in this way from taking responsibility for their actions. Second, the presumed aim of such a programme is to encourage men to say no to fucking. More preferable is a programme, open to all and not only to the feeble-minded few, which validates, explicates and empowers individuals in a range of circumstances to choose whether or not to fuck.

It is no accident that relapse emerges as a problem in the AIDS literature as funding for AIDS prevention work is becoming scarcer, and particularly as the process of the 'de-gaying' of AIDS gathers pace. It was doubtless seen as a way to re-establish the needs of gay men in the fight for scarce resources. While understandable, the idea is fundamentally misguided in that it reinforces a discourse of gay men as incapable, deficient victims of circumstance. The current lack of funding for health promotion initiatives for gay and bisexual men is justified because gay men are supposed to have 'got their act together': to have made the changes in sexual behaviour necessary in the face of this appalling pandemic. It is, however, naïve to believe that an acceptance by decision-makers of the notion of relapse will lead to funds becoming suddenly and miraculously available. If relapse is accepted, we face the chilling likelihood that funds will not be forthcoming because we are irresponsible, feckless and deserve all we get. Such a prospect should, with Hamlet, give us pause 'and [make] us rather bear those ills we have/ than fly to others that we know not of.'

Notes

1 At present Project SIGMA is Paul Broderick, Tony Coxon, Peter Davies, Ford Hickson, Andrew Hunt, Tom McManus, Michael Stephens and Peter Weatherburn.

2   The term 'unsafe sex' is used deliberately but with considerable unease: there seem to be almost as many definitions of 'unsafe' or 'risky' behaviour as there are papers talking about it. At the recent International Conference on AIDS held in Florence, definitions included such items as visiting a prostitute, having more than one partner, visiting an STD clinic.

3   The view is widely held, especially among non-American researchers. See Baxter (1990), Hart *et al.* (1992), Bochow (1991).

References

ADIB, S.M., JOSEPH, J.G., OSTROW, D.G., TAL, M. and SCHWARTZ, S.M. (1991) 'Relapse in Sexual Behaviour among Homosexual Men: A Two-year Follow-up from the Chicago MACS/CCS', *AIDS*, 5, pp. 757–60.

AJZEN, I. and MADDEN, T.J. (1986) 'Prediction of Goal-Directed Behavior: Attitudes, Intentions and Perceived Behavioral Control', *Journal of Experimental Social Psychology*, 22, pp. 453–74.

BAXTER, D. (1990) 'Maintenance of Safe Sex Norms in the Gay Community', Paper presented at the Fourth Australian National AIDS Conference, Canberra.

BOCHOW, M. (1991) 'Le Safer Sex, "Une Discussion sans Fin"': Quelques Remarques au Sujet de la Discussion Actuelle', in M. POLLAK (Ed.), *Homosexualités et SIDA*, Paris, Caille Gai-Kitsch-Camp.

CATANIA, J.A., KEGELES, S.M. and COATES, T.J. (19) 'Towards an Understanding of Risk Behaviour: The CAPS AIDS Risk Reduction Model (ARRM)', *Health Education Quarterly*, 17, pp. 53–72.

DAVIES, P.M. and WEATHERBURN, P. (1991) 'Towards a General Model of Sexual Negotiation', in P. AGGLETON, G. HART and P.M. DAVIES (Eds), *AIDS: Responses, Interventions and Care*, Lewes, Falmer Press.

DAVIES, P.M., HUNT, A.J., MACOURT, M.P.A. and WEATHERBURN, P. (1990) *A Longitudinal Study of the Sexual Behaviour of Homosexual Males under the Impact of AIDS: A Final Report to the Department of Health*, London, Project SIGMA.

EKSTRAND, M.L., STALL, R.D., COATES, T.J. and MCKUSICK, L. (1989) 'Risky Sex Relapse, the Next Challenge for AIDS Prevention Programs: The AIDS Behavioural Research Project', Paper presented at Fifth International Conference on AIDS, Montreal.

FITZPATRICK, R., BOULTON, M. and HART, G. (1989) 'Gay Men's Sexual Behaviour in Response to AIDS', in P. AGGLETON, G., HART and P.M., DAVIES (Eds), *AIDS: Social Representations, Social Practices*, Lewes, Falmer Press.

HART, G., *et al.*, (1992) 'Relapse to Unsafe Sexual Behaviour amongst Gay Men: a critique of recent behavioural HNIAIDS research', *Sociology of Health and Illness*, 14, pp. 216–232.

JELLINEK, E.M. (1960) *The Disease Concept of Alcoholism*, New Haven, Conn., Hillhouse.

POLLAK, M. (1988) *Les Homosexuels et le SIDA: Sociologie d'une Epidemie*, Paris, A.M. Metailie.

PRIEUR, A. (1990) 'Gay Men: Reasons for Continued Practice of Unsafe Sex', *AIDS Education and Prevention*, 2, 2, pp. 110–17.

ROSENSTOCK, K. (1974) 'The Health Belief Model and Preventive Health Behaviour', *Health Education Monograph*, 2, pp. 354–65.

SHERR, L. and STRONG, C. (1990) 'Can Safe Sex be Maintained? A Study of Relapse', Paper presented at the British Psychological Society London Conference.

STALL, R.D., EKSTRAND, M., POLLACK, L., MCKUSICK, L. and COATES, T. (1990) 'Relapse to Unsafe Sex: the next challenge for AIDS prevention efforts', *Journal of Acquired Immunodeficiency Syndrome*, 3, 12, pp. 1181–1187.

11 Pressure, Resistance, Empowerment: Young Women and the Negotiation of Safer Sex

Janet Holland, Caroline Ramazanoglu, Sue Scott, Sue Sharpe and Rachel Thomson

Knowledge of the risks concerning the sexual transmission of HIV among young heterosexuals is spreading, but controlling sexual safety can be problematic for young women if they play subordinate roles in sexual encounters. Once people have been given information on how HIV can be transmitted sexually, and advice on safer sex, they still have to make sense of what they have learned. They have to consider whether what they know has any bearing on their own lives, and how, when or whether to put this knowledge into practice. Rates of teenage pregnancy and rising rates of sexually transmitted disease indicate that, whatever women's intentions, risky sexual practices are still widespread among young heterosexuals (OPCS, 1991; Estaugh and Wheatley, 1990).

Previous research in medical sociology indicates that possession of knowledge has no necessary connection with changes in risk-taking behaviour (Azjen and Fishbein, 1980; Hanson *et al.*, 1987). Knowledge of risk has to be incorporated into people's understandings of their own situations to bring about any interest in change, and this involves people in an active process of reflection (Raven and Litman-Adizes, 1986; Hunt and Macleod, 1987). Such knowledge as does exist at present about the behaviour of heterosexuals indicates little change to safer sexual behaviour, apart from a slightly increased use of condoms (*AIDS Newsletter*, 10 December 1990). Department of Health figures in January 1991 show that while new cases of HIV seropositivity in gay and bisexual men fell between 1989 and the end of 1990, new cases of seropositive heterosexual men and women increased over the same period. Current projections show the proportion of seropositive women to men is likely to increase steadily (OPCS, 1991).

We have argued previously (Holland *et al.*, 1991a) that variations in levels of power and autonomy in the negotiation of sexual encounters can contribute to unsafe sexual behaviour. Young women have to cope with conflicting social pressures in organizing their sexual behaviour and the outcomes can be both positive and negative. The extent to which young heterosexual women define sex in terms of love, romance and relationships with men, leads to a widespread acceptance of sexual practices being defined in terms of men's needs. This gives men, whether wittingly or not, considerable power over young women's sexual practices. The tragedy of the AIDS epidemic has now given urgency to questions about the ways in which safer sexual practices can be promoted within gendered social relationships.

Women who want to ensure their own sexual safety have to be socially assertive and prepared to challenge, to some extent at least, the conventions of femininity (Holland *et al.*, 1991a). Those who value their control of sexuality have to be prepared to lose the valued social relationship with a sexual partner or potential partner (see also Gross and Bellew-Smith, 1983). Young women who assert their own needs have to negotiate sexual relationships with men which resist the common sense of masculine and feminine sexuality. The understanding of sexual risk-taking by young women and the promotion of safer sex for young heterosexuals will depend on how we can make connections between the sexual pressures on young women, their resistance to these pressures and their personal empowerment in managing their own lives.

In this chapter we reflect on the sexual politics of safer sex by considering the ways in which the empowerment of young women can be conceptualized in sexual encounters.[1] These related themes of pressure, resistance and empowerment are developed through analysis of data from the Women, Risk and AIDS Project's interviews with 150 young women in London and Manchester.[2] From these young women's accounts of their sexual relationships, we consider the question of how far their needs for sexual safety are compromised by pressures to service men's needs in sexual relationships, and how far they subordinate their own sexual safety to their expectations of men's needs and desires. We argue that for a young woman to negotiate safe sex in a heterosexual relationship she has to be empowered both to develop a positive conception of feminine sexuality and able to put this positive conception into practice. We argue below that empowerment at one level does not necessarily entail empowerment at another.

The Context of Empowerment: Pressures from Men in Sexual Encounters

Most of the young women's accounts of their first sexual experiences are either negative or indicate limited satisfaction. When young women, often under the age of consent, begin to engage in sexual relationships and to test their sexual identities, they do not initially have direct personal experience to draw on, and much that they need to know is hidden from them.[3] They have to make sense of information from different sources — childhood experiences, schools, youth workers, parents and siblings, peers, the mass media — which often give them contradictory messages (Thompson, 1984). Since there is no overriding conception of a positive and enjoyable female sexuality in which women are both acceptably feminine and in control of their sexuality, they have to relate the ideas about love, romance and femininity, which they bring to their sexual relationships, to their initial experiences with men.

Nearly a quarter of the sample (thirty-five young women out of 150) had had unwanted sexual intercourse in response to pressure from men.[4] These pressures varied from mild insistence on giving way to intercourse or to intercourse on his terms, to threats, physical assault, child abuse and rape. Young women in their interviews gave accounts of situations in which various forms of violence had played a part and in which they had to make sense of the extent to which they could exercise control over their own sexuality. Even where women had not been directly pressured by men, or were not sexually active, the extent to which male pressure is incorporated into the conventions of 'normal' heterosexuality provides the cultural context within which young women have to negotiate their own safety (Hanmer and Maynard, 1987; Kelly, 1988; Stanko, 1985). Health promotion strategies then need to take this context of pressure into account.

Safer Sex, Heterosexuality and the Empowerment of Young Women

In the health promotion literature there is little or no account of gendered power relations which could challenge conceptions of heterosexual sex as natural. There has been a tendency for the Health Education Authority and other producers of educational materials in the UK to focus on a narrow conception of heterosexuality which is drawn in a male image. The senior programme officer for the HEA's Sexual Health Programme has commented: '. . . our advertising directed at heterosexuals has necessarily concentrated on the need for protected penetrative sex' (Christophers, 1990).

It is significant that while the AIDS crisis has opened up a possibility of validating non-penetrative sexual practices, and thus of a move towards less male-centred understandings of heterosexuality (Coward, 1987), the dominant definition of safer sex has focused on how to reduce the risks attached to vaginal penetration. The success of this definition can be illustrated by the fact that the majority of our respondents equated safer sex simply and directly with condom use. Heterosexual sexuality continues to be closely tied at the level of ideology to procreation; any move towards separating sex from reproduction leads to anxiety and outrage as is evidenced by the 'virgin birth' debate (Rumbold, 1991).

Thinking about empowerment in relation to safer sex is constrained by existing assumptions and categories of thought which define heterosexual sex in terms of a dominant masculinity. This conception of heterosexuality tends to perceive safer sex as the responsibility of individual men and women who are free to make rational choices for their own protection. The logical consequence of this rational choice model of sexual action has been to direct sex education towards individuals in order to inform their choices (Jessop and Thorogood, 1989).[5] It leaves as unproblematic the conception of sex as a set of acts leading to penetration and male orgasm. In this conception of sex, safety becomes reduced to the punctual intervention of the condom (Freeman and Scott, 1990). Young women's knowledge of and access to contraception may effectively structure what is thought of as 'sex'. The definition of safer sex in terms of effective condom use reinforces, through practice, the central place of male erection and orgasm in sexual encounters. To plan to protect oneself with a condom presupposes something to put it on.[6] Condoms should not be seen as a neutral and rational response to HIV prevention, but as a compromise with existing partriarchal ideology and practices. The extent to which the nature of heterosexuality is assumed leaves, as Wilton and Aggleton (1990) have put it, 'heterosexual man as the great undiscussed'.

Mukesh Kapila suggests that:

> In the long term, a sexually healthy population requires the creation of a social climate which enables individuals to relate to each other in mutually respectful relationships. Only then will individual-directed education be acceptable . . . we can't expect all individuals to solve problems which really belong in a wider context. (Williams, 1990)

The point which Kapila overlooks is that heterosexual relationships do not take place between socially equivalent individuals but between gendered persons. The practical problems of how 'mutually respectful relationships' can emerge from the inequalities of gender have still to be addressed. The conception of safer sex as a matter of individual choice and responsibility separates it from debates about citizenship which could place sexual safety on a public and collective agenda alongside such issues as child abuse, violence against women and new reproductive technologies. It is not yet the case that the promotion of safer sex has been wholly medicalized; rather, it is currently a contested terrain in which safer heterosexual identities can be negotiated in struggle against the idea of natural and dominant male sexuality.

In considering the implications of our data, we consider it important to evaluate critically the 'solutions' to HIV/AIDS which have come from state agencies and biomedicine. The perceived need for an absolute guide to safety has rendered health promotion dependent on imperfect medical knowledge about the different kinds of risks. The hidden assumption in many safer sex guidelines (Setters, 1988) is that decisions about risk in relation to HIV are governed by rationality, rather than by the multi-faceted and often contradictory pressures of everyday life.

If we want to think of women as able to struggle against the pressures of patriarchal societies, by finding their own sources of power, we need to be specific as to what these sources could be. While some young women are relatively advantaged by their class background, their level of education or their ethnicity, there is no clear material or gendered base for sexual empowerment. It is easy to talk of how to empower young women so as to make sex safer or more pleasurable; it is harder to specify what exactly is meant by empowerment in relation to safer sex. There is a tension here between ideas of empowerment as individual assertiveness or individual choice, and a more collective notion of empowerment as a challenge to dominant masculinity. Whereas the exercise of male power is taken to be the subordination and control of women by men, we do not take women's empowerment to be the subordination of men.

Envisaging empowerment for young women means defining the power relations which could be changed and defining how these relationships can be transformed. In the context of sexual encounters, empowering women could mean: not engaging in sexual activity; not engaging in sexual activity without informed consent; getting men to consent to safer practices; negotiating sexual practices which are pleasurable to women as well as to men.

The Method of Analysis

To clarify what empowerment means in practice, we have used the technique of systemic networks in the analysis of our data.[7] The use of the network allows us to organize our data in terms of a range of sources of pressure from men and the empowerment of young women. This gives us a theoretical map of the pressures and responses which impinge on young women's sexuality. The empowerment network which we have used for this chapter is laid out in Figure 1,[8] and the young women's accounts which follow have been analyzed using the categories in this network. For the purposes of this chapter, we consider only the key categories to show, through young women's accounts, how empowerment can be understood as a process of struggle, rather then as a static category of knowledge or practice.

In coding and analyzing the interview transcripts in terms of this network, we drew on three levels of conceptualization: the terms and meanings used by the young women and explicit in the data; the interviewer's fieldnotes made after the interview, which entail some interpretation of meanings in the interview; team members' discussion, interpretation and coding of these data in the light of feminist and sociological theory.[9] These levels of interpretation helped us to analyze accounts of pressure and empowerment where the researchers' interpretation differed from that of the young women: for example, where a young woman defined herself as empowered, and the researchers did not want to categorize her in this way. The interaction of these levels of interpretation is built into the categories of the network.

This network is based on the analysis of a sub-set of twenty-six young women whose accounts identified them as relatively empowered in negotiations around sexual intercourse and sexual relationships. Of these, twenty-two were or had been sexually active, and eleven of these, that is half of those who were sexually active, had had pressured sexual experiences in the form of sexual abuse as children, rape or unwanted sexual intercourse under threat or other pressure from men. In comparison with the sample as whole, this sub-set of twenty-six was very slightly biased towards the middle class and the older age groups. They had, on average, slightly more casual sexual partners than the sample as a whole. Fifteen had had unprotected sex which had put them at potential risk of HIV infection, and eight had had unprotected sex which put them at risk of pregnancy, but this was a lower rate of unsafe sex than that of the sample as a whole. In other respects they did not differ significantly from the rest of the sample.

To bring out the main points of this analysis, we discuss the cases of five young women whose accounts illustrate different aspects of the contradictory processes of empowerment.

Empowerment as Process

The empowerment network is not conceptualized as a set of static categories to which young women can be assigned, but as a way of capturing the processes and possibilities of women's attempts to gain control of their sexuality. The empowerment of young women in negotiating safer sexual encounters can never simply be achieved but must be constantly struggled for.

The strategies for safer sex which young women bring to their sexual relationships help to shape the ways in which they plan sexual relationships and sexual practices. Their initial experiences have to be made sense of in terms of the actual outcomes of sexual encounters, which may differ considerably from their

Figure 1   A Model of Women's Empowerment in Relation to Sexuality, Sexual Encounters and Relationships

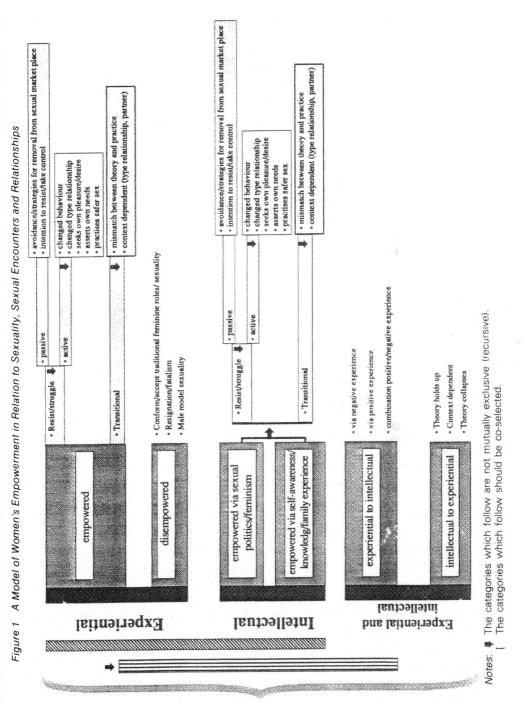

Notes: ➡ The categories which follow are not mutually exclusive (recursive).
[The categories which follow should be co-selected.

intentions. Making sense of this gap can then affect how empowered they may be in future relationships.

Since knowledge, intentions and control of situations in practice are not necessarily congruent, we have conceptualized young women's behaviour in terms of two levels. The *intellectual level* is that of the knowledge, expectations and intentions they bring to an encounter. The *experiential level* is the level of their sexual practice. The relationship between the intellectual and the experiential is never static, but develops and changes over time, as young women try to bring expectations and control of sexual situations more closely together. While empowerment always depends on gaining men's consent to women's definitions of the terms of sexual encounters, effective strategies for safer sex do not seem possible without some congruence between the intellectual and the experiential levels of empowerment.

Central to our understanding of empowerment is a third concept, that of a transitional level in the network. Since the empowerment of young women in sexual encounters is unstable and struggled over, the transitional category indicates that women may be empowered to the extent of controlling sexual encounters in some situations or with some partners, but not in others or with subsequent partners. This context-specific empowerment gives us a transitional rather than a static category. This notion of transition is an attempt to identify situations in which there is a mismatch between young women's intellectual empowerment and their capacity to put their intentions of controlling their sexuality into practice.

Young women can move in or out of this category in a process of interaction between intellectual and experiential levels of empowerment, with different outcomes in different sexual encounters, or over time. The additional category of the combined intellectual/experiential level is a further attempt to grasp the process.

Intellectual Empowerment

The problem of trying to classify young women according to their state of empowerment is illustrated by the category of intellectual empowerment. Both negative and positive sexual experiences can lead to empowerment in the form of self-awareness or knowledge based on the broader implications of sexual politics. But empowerment at the intellectual level is not sufficient to ensure safer sex. Young women who are empowered at this level may have sexual experiences which they are not able to control or resist, pushing them back into the transitional category where they have to struggle to gain ground that had been attained only at an intellectual level.

A number of young women expressed powerful intentions in their interviews: they gave accounts of their understanding of the risks of sexual encounters and of their intentions in future sexual encounters. It was not possible in a single interview to follow up these intentions, but in those cases where young women reported retrospectively on their intentions and subsequent experiences the problems of putting intentions into practice were discussed. This came out clearly in cases where women understood the risks of unprotected sexual intercourse and intended to use condoms for their own safety, but in practice did not do so (Holland *et al.*, 1991a). A 20 per cent sub-sample of young women have been interviewed for a second time and, in Nicky's case, the problems of treating intellectual empowerment as a static category can be seen in her account of her experiences between her first and second interviews.

Nicky[10]

Nicky was an attractive, confident young woman, not sexually active at our first interview, but very clear as to what her requirements would be of a partner. She was both very knowledgeable and concerned about HIV and AIDS and, when asked if she would take precautions in that respect if she were to have a sexual relationship, she asserted:

> N: Yeah, well if I wouldn't then I wouldn't be in a relationship with them — I wouldn't if they couldn't accept that. It's just mindless not to be aware of the risks and prepared to lessen them now.

Nicky can be regarded as intellectually empowered on several grounds: family background and support; personal conviction and self-awareness; the ideology and practice of feminism and sexual politics. But the limitations of intellectual empowerment were demonstrated in the second interview, which illustrated the processes involved in gaining and attempting to retain empowerment. Nicky had by then had three sexual relationships, and although she had mostly been able to uphold her insistence on safer sex, she had had unprotected sex on a number of occasions. She described her first experience of sex as good, although she was drunk at the time and unprotected. She took the morning after pill. After this it was usually condoms, 'nasty little things, a bit revolting really, but worth it'. This first boyfriend had been violent, although she presents this as shared violence despite some voiced doubts:

> N: We used to beat each other up quite frequently, every other day. . . . It does sound really bizarre and horrible, but it was quite enjoyable in a funny sort of way. We both used to call a truce before we did any real damage. I have got bruises. I had bruises for the entire [time of the relationship].

> N: I think if I'd wanted to stop it, I would have done. I remember, thinking, 'this is really strange'. But I didn't — I'm not a violent person, I never fight. It seemed almost that he needed — he needed that, and in a way when he needed that, I went along with it.

The fights usually ended in sex, although the sex 'was always him. It was for him. It wasn't really for me. He — he used to, you know, just get on with it really.' After this sexual relationship finished, in a rather complicated fashion, the boyfriend visited her and effectively raped her, by forcing her to have sex which she did not want — she felt used and abused but could not stop him. She thought he had interpreted the event differently from her, since he had a notion of their relationship as one in which they could not control themselves. She had a scare about pregnancy at this point.

The second relationship 'was actually completely sexual. I mean, I was going out with him for four months, and I never once saw him in daylight', but the sex was a lot better. This particular relationship demonstrated elements of the 'male model of sexuality', since she saw their mutual interest being in a non-committed, non-involved sexual relationship, in which they could each have other partners. It ended when the young man went abroad. She subsequently embarked on what she took to be a serious relationship, only to be dropped by the young man without warning or explanation.

The start of Nicky's sexual relationships illustrated the movement from intellectual empowerment to sexual experiences in which it was difficult to maintain that power. In some respects she did, in that she was usually, although clearly not always, able to practise safer sex. She maintained a stance of equality in relationships, taking the first sexual partner with her to the clinic to get the morning after pill, but in many respects she was vulnerable and even abused, unable to stop unprotected sex being physically forced upon her, unable to protect herself emotionally from being abandoned by a sexual partner. 'Mug, mug', was her own comment on herself.

The Struggle for Empowerment: The Male Model

While a number of young women gave accounts of their assertiveness in relation to men, much of this behaviour was not empowering in practice. The male model stresses the freedom of the individual to engage in sexual relationships without personal obligation. This disguises inequalities of power and control in sexual relationships with a liberal discourse of personal choice. It is an attractive model of sexual empowerment for young women who are trying to take control of their own lives and are resisting a passive model of female sexuality, but it does not allow women to recognize or challenge male power.

The case which follows is of a young women who is consciously trying to be sexually empowered, to operate sexually on an equal basis with men. However, the way in which she conceives her empowerment is contradicted by her involvement in relationships where her sexual practice puts her at risk.

Angela

At the time of her interview Angela was 18 years old. She was supposed to be attending college, had her own car and, in her words, was 'totally going out in search of a good time.' She had recently become involved in a punk scene based in a council estate in which drug use, including injecting drug use, was common. She was four weeks into a relationship with Tony whom she described as 'a bit of a drop out'. For Angela, who had had a conventional middle-class upbringing, this new life was challenging and exciting. She perceived herself as empowered by the choices she was making as part of her personal growth.

A: I am not trying to shock them [parents and old friends] but I'm just trying to find myself and find out what sort of person I really am. I just do what I want to do because I don't want to get older and wish I had done that when I was younger. I intend doing it when I am younger so I have got no regrets.

Her aspirations in terms of sexual relationships show a similar confidence and a desire to engage on equal terms with men, challenging conventional models of feminine behaviour.

> A: I just get carried away. I believe in equality, like a woman has a need as much as a man, and I think at the time, 'Oh yes, sod it'. A fellow is allowed to get a pat on the back and a drink bought them.

This male model of sexual assertiveness includes a belief in her right to sexual pleasure.

> A: If a man is going with a woman he gets his pleasure, and then it's wrong that a lot of lads don't bother so much about the woman. Sort of like a quick grope then in and out sort of thing and I hate that. I think you have got to have consideration. With this lad — that I think was one of the most pleasurable experiences I ever had. But I think it is pretty important to a woman, we're entitled to it.

However, this assertiveness, which can be conceived as intellectual empowerment, is experienced in a rather contradictory way. First, she is attracted to men who will be a challenge to her, including men who will have power over her. She commented on a previous partner:

> A: I hate weak men. He would do anything [I wanted him to] and I hate that. So I want someone who will keep me in my place.

Despite her intellectual empowerment, in her sexual practice she does not necessarily find herself able to act according to her intentions or to control sexual situations.

> A: Sometimes you feel dead guilty when you are with a lad and [have] not tried to get him turned on and you feel it hard and pressed against your leg, and you're thinking 'Oh shit, I didn't want that to happen at all.' When I was younger I used to think I'll just let him, because I didn't want to be known as a prick tease.

In practice she experiences vulnerability.

> A: I think I've got a bit of a muddle up somewhere along the line, because I interpret sex as feeling — well, if I feel unwanted and then I sleep with him then it makes me feel wanted. I was thinking last night and saying to him 'I've gone wrong somewhere' because I shouldn't have to do that.

Angela first had intercourse at 15. Initially she relied on occasional condom use combined with taking chances. Her best friend who relied purely on luck became pregnant and eventually had an abortion. This event provided an opportunity for Angela to reflect on her own behaviour. Making a decision to go on the pill, despite fear of her mother finding out, can be seen as an empowering practice on the young woman's part and part of her growing assertiveness.

Although she had practised safer sex episodically in the past by using condoms, once she was using the pill she had to think more deliberately about risk-taking in sexual encounters. When asked about her intentions in relation to the practice of safer sex she recognized this.

> *A:* If I met a lad who I didn't know anything about, I wouldn't think, well I'm on the pill and that will do, I think I would use a condom.

However, subsequent discussion of her present relationship revealed putting safer sex into practice to be rather more problematic.

> *A:* Tony doesn't really like using them. That used to annoy me, the fact that he knew we were going out and that we would probably end up [having sex without a condom].

Although she felt that asking a man to use a condom as a contraceptive was acceptable, citing fear of HIV as a reason was less easy.

> *A:* I think that they would probably be dead insulted . . . I would take it personally, I would feel insulted.

The pill allows women to engage with men sexually without depending on them for contraception. Being on the pill allows women to meet men's needs without challenging the power dimension of the sexual situation. If a woman asks a man to use a condom when she is already on the pill, this alters the balance of the relationship by bringing into question the nature of the relationship and recognizing the independent rights of both of those involved.

Angela's interview indicated the vulnerability of her position with Tony. Having said that she felt that AIDS only affected so-called 'risk groups', she goes on to reveal that Tony has not only been injecting intravenously for two years but at times sharing needles, and that they do not have safer sex. Despite her intention of remaining in control of her sexual practice, her empowerment at the experiential level is undermined by the complicated issues of trust and commitment in this relationship.

> *A:* He always goes on about I don't trust him but when it comes down to it I think I do trust him, like I know he wouldn't go with anyone else, because he is a sort of one woman man, whereas I am like not a one man woman.

Angela's use of the contraceptive pill can be interpreted in terms of a male model of sexual empowerment. This model can be intellectually empowering, but is not empowering at the experiential level. The contradiction between the theory and practice of sexual empowerment is sharply focused by the risks she takes in having unsafe sex with Tony. Angela copes with these contradictions between intention and practice by distancing herself from the risks of HIV.

> *A:* I don't know anyone who has got AIDS so it's not too hard to forget about it.

Context-specific Empowerment:
The Constraints on Experiential Empowerment

Sarah

Unlike Angela, Sarah was having safer sex at the time of her interview, in the sense that she was in a supposedly monogamous relationship and both she and her boyfriend had had HIV tests before the relationship became sexual. This situation was initiated by Sarah in that she felt herself to have been at risk in previous relationships and had suggested the tests. She indicates a process of self-reflection from which self-awareness develops, leading to a need to take control of her sexuality; a process that we can understand as intellectual empowerment. However, as she herself points out, such empowerment does not change the social world.

> S: . . . we have all these things on paper, all these theories where we say 'yes, we do this' but when it comes down to it would we do it? Have we done it? I think it takes quite a long time to develop. You can't just suddenly discover things and say 'yes I will behave like that in future', you can't do that, you have to work towards it.

Sarah has managed to control and order events in such a way that she does feel in control of her present sexual relationship, but she acknowledges that she could be vulnerable again in the future:

> S: I was telling myself, if this relationship comes to an end, I'm never falling in the same trap as before, I'll make sure that I won't . . . I'm more than 50 per cent confident that I won't, but not a full 100 per cent.

The story which Sarah told in the interview is marked by a recognition of her powerlessness and vulnerability in previous relationships and a dissatisfaction with the quality of those relationships. The trauma of an unplanned pregnancy, subsequent abortion and a cervical cancer scare appears to have acted as a catalyst enabling her to redefine her sexual behaviour and identity. However, her explanation of this change is somewhat contradictory. On one hand she employs the restrictive discourse of post-AIDS morality to condemn the kind of sexual relationship and the model of sexual morality in which she was previously involved:

> S: You see the adverts on the media all the time telling you that it is bad to have so many sexual partners and that is why you have got all these increases — AIDS, and this is why there's an increase in cervical cancer in people under 25 and all this. . . . I think at the beginning I was thinking that it was normal, then I suddenly had this backlash when I thought it was a really bad thing that I had done by sleeping with these people.

On the other hand, we find that her rejection of this male model of sexual empowerment is rooted in her recognition of her own experience of powerlessness within such relationships. Her argument focuses upon a critical interpretation of the concept of choice:

> S: I thought it was that you had more choice, but I really wasn't having any choice in the matter. It's like the whole thing of the sixties, that sex is free for all. More of it available for more men, there is no risk in it. At the time I hadn't realized that was the case, that you had to decide, not just go along with it because it seems to be alright.

This growing awareness of her own powerlessness to decide and control the shape of her sexual relationships is reflected in her recollections of past behaviour.

> S: It wasn't that I wanted to take control over the other person, I just wanted to take an active part — I wasn't — I would be constantly doing things I didn't want to, and afterwards I would be chastising myself — I didn't realize why, but if there was someone there who would say, 'yes, come out with me', I could say, 'no'. But then if there was some physical contact then I couldn't say no. . . . It took me a long time to work out that these were the situations where I had a lack of power.

Available models of appropriate 'feminine' sexuality, which value passivity, place young women at a particular disadvantage when they are engaging with men on the basis of a male-defined model of sexual empowerment and sexual norms.

> S: . . . there was one particular relationship where I was sleeping with someone and I thought I was having a relationship, but they didn't know that they were having a relationship. Like that type of thing. It kept getting worse.

> S: I let myself get into a situation where I wasn't in control. I'm never doing it again. I'm going to sort it all out now for good.

For Sarah, making an active decision to enter a new relationship was an expression of self-awareness and in itself a strategy of intellectual empowerment.

> S: I also didn't start seeing him for a long time you know for — it was just after I had had an abortion and things like that. I didn't want to see anybody, and I didn't want to just fall into the thing you know, 'if he likes me it will do, it doesn't matter you know, what you feel', so I left it for a long time, about four months or something and didn't see him, and I actually decided to go into the relationship, not just sort of went along with it, I decided, and it is an active decision-making relationship instead of just jogging along.

The degree of control and responsibility which women exercise within sexual relationships has always been structured by their fears of pregnancy. The process of empowerment is structured in part by their experiences of and attitudes towards these contraceptive responsibilities. The additional necessity of safe sex, be it condom use, non-penetrative sex and/or monogamy, has further complicated this. Empowerment cannot simply be equated with safe sex. For Sarah, deciding to stop taking the pill was initially a positive and empowering decision.

> S: I had decided that I did not want to take the pill, because I didn't see why I should take something internally and mess up my body when he could use a condom.

But condom use is problematic in that in necessitates a direct confrontation with male power within a sensitive and often non-verbal context.

> S: I mean it is alright to think in advance — to use a condom all the time, but when it comes down to it either you won't or maybe you will. And that is what happened then — I didn't. It was a complete mistake, so I decided I would never let it happen again . . . because with a condom it is still your responsibility in a way, but then you are not wholly in control of it.

For these reasons Sarah returned to using the pill: 'I would rather rely on myself than anyone else.' Both she and her boyfriend had an HIV test and Sarah takes their relationship to be monogamous.

Sarah's account indicates some of the complexity of bringing intellectual and experiential levels of empowerment together. While clearly intellectually empowered, she recognized situations where she could be at risk despite understanding and awareness. To ensure that she is in sexual relationships in which she can exercise control, Sarah would have to be experientially empowered in a more stable way than she indicated in her interview. This does not mean being confident that she can always take control, nor that she could manage safer sex in any sexual situation. Rather, it entails recognizing situations where she can be both intellectually and experientially empowered and avoiding situations within which she would be vulnerable.

Context-specific empowerment is a transitional and unstable category. This form of empowerment can lead to safer sex, for example, through lying to a partner about being on the pill and using condoms as well, or as Sarah did, having an HIV test and then maintaining a monogamous relationship. However, it remains a limited form of empowerment; women may control particular situations, but they do so without seriously confronting male power, and so their strategies for safer sex may not always work.

Intellectual/Experiential Empowerment

Sharon

Sharon's sexual career had been a particularly negative and pressured set of experiences. Her account illustrates a painful process of developing self-knowledge and a conscious attempt to marry her intellectual empowerment, or what she thinks of as her bravery, to her control of her sexuality. The fragility of her level of empowerment indicates both the possibilities of women's resistance to men's pressures and the depth of critical reflection on their experience which women need to become empowered.

The event Sharon initially defined as her first sexual experiences was being raped at a school party when she was fourteen.

> Q: When you were first raped did you understand it as rape?
> Sh: No. I mean I could say now it was a rape, but even still — there's still doubts in my mind. I keep thinking to myself, I was drunk.

She did, however, remember her response in terms of resistance.

> Sh: ...I can remember screaming, and I can remember someone shouting something — and I can remember him running off... I can remember running....

When she was older she had a sexual relationship with a man who physically assaulted her. She left him, then went back to him, even though he had threatened her with a knife and, after escaping again, had been pursued by letters, phone calls and threats. She described the pressure to have sex in this relationship:

> Sh: I wouldn't say he was good in bed, or he didn't do anything for me anyway. But there was no night went by without it, because that's the way he wanted it. If I didn't have it he was a total shit.
> Q: Were you able to say what you wanted, that you didn't want to have sex?
> Sh: If I didn't want to have sex there would have been violence.

Sharon shows that young women can actively resist men's power, even when this power is exercised violently, but their resistance may not necessarily be very effective. Sharon had not just resisted, but had also reflected on her experiences and on what she wanted. In a subsequent relationship she gave an account of herself as much more assertive. She had consciously decided to specify her own needs in the relationship.

> Sh: Tonight we were supposed to be going out on our own for the evening, and we're not. We're not because he's made different plans. So I turned round and I told him 'OK tonight we'll do what you want, Friday we'll do what I want.' So I'm brave enough to do that now....

This progression between pressured sex and empowerment in Sharon's understanding of her experiences indicates the complexities of understanding empowerment. Towards the end of this interview Sharon mentioned that in the last few months she had come to recognize that she had been sexually abused as a child, 'Oh, the police were involved in it and everything, but I just couldn't admit to myself that it was abuse.' This exploration of her past sexuality had altered her understanding of female sexuality.

Q: Did you expect to enjoy sex at that time?

Sh: No, no. Now I'm learning it can be. I've still not found it, but . . .! I mean. I know it's possible now to actually enjoy it, you know, and get full pleasure out of it. I've just got to figure out how to do it.

She went on to say that she had never had an orgasm, and that her next step was to get to know her current boyfriend before starting a sexual relationship, in the hope of learning to find pleasure in sex.

Sh: . . . emotionally I feel like a virgin. I feel like I've yet to experience sex. All I've ever had is the physical side, now I want the emotional side.

We have conceptualized Sharon as both intellectually and experientially empowered at the time of her interview in that she has identified pressure as coming from men and from her own experiences of sexual violence. For from being a victim, she envisages herself as having agency. The changes in her knowledge and expectations enabled her to exercise control in her current relationship.

Tina

Tina illustrated a much more assured process of integrating intellectual and experiential levels of empowerment since she had learned that men had to be educated if women were to ensure their own sexual safety and sexual pleasure.

At the time of this interview Tina was 21 years old, living independently from her family and unemployed. She had left home at 18, feeling that she had escaped from a difficult family (her mother died of cervical cancer when she was 15 and father subsequently remarried) and from a poor working-class neighbourhood. She was very aware of the social pressures and constraints of the area in which she grew up. This type of social awareness was matched by a strong assertion of personal agency, a quality which she ascribed to the influence of her mother.

This sense of agency is reflected in her discussion of her experiences of relationships in the past. Her first sexual experience was with another woman, after which she went out with older boys 'probably because a lot of boys my age were emotionally immature'. However, her confidence is matched by an awareness of the way in which power is embedded in many forms of sexual relationships and a willingness to confront this power.

T: I saw friends, people I know, go out with older blokes and being frightened to say no, or to suggest things — because the bloke would be older. And they didn't feel fully in control of their own bodies — feelings like what was an orgasm? Most women didn't know what they should feel. It was very much on the receiving side, doing something to please someone else. Not pleasure for themselves. So when it came down to contraception, 'Oh I went on the pill to please my boyfriend', because they didn't like sheaths for whatever reason. They didn't feel in control, as an equal, with the same rights as their boyfriend, because they were younger.

In her contraceptive practice this young woman was a health educator's dream. Her first sexual experience which included intercourse with a man was seen as positive, planned and protected. Using a condom was a 'mutual decision'. She subsequently went on to the pill while continuing to use condoms. Her sexual practice in her relationships was informed by a shrewd understanding of practical sexual politics and a willingness to engage in confrontation.

> *T:* A lot of men don't actually realize that you do have pleasure out of it. Or that you should. Or they're so engrossed in what they're doing or feeling that you don't come into it at all.

Her experience went beyond confrontation into negotiation over sexual practice in which, unlike Angela who had been afraid of being labelled a prick tease, Tina thought that men should think about what they were doing.

> *T:* In a blackmail situation where a boy's got an erection and he wants to have sexual intercourse with me, I don't. Then I'll talk about it and start laughing. I'll say 'look what you're doing, it's totally unreasonable'. I'll put the funny side on to it. Get them to actually think about what they're doing. Because the majority of men don't think — 'well why am I doing this?' There's a lot of people who did things they didn't really want to do. So I'm thinking, well why did they do it? Through thinking about things like that, everyday things, so [now] I can discuss things with people which are of a delicate nature. I've got over it, but I did go through it. I haven't always been able to say 'No, no I don't', 'no I won't.'

Tina had been able to integrate the theory and practice of empowerment in an unusually strong way. Such integration relies on both a pragmatic understanding of, and a positive response to, the 'masculinist' rules of sexual interaction. By valuing her own sense of self and independence she is able to define her own version of sexual practice. In heterosexual sexual interaction this, by definition, entails engaging with men and a male model of sexual practice.

When asked about her sexual behaviour in the context of HIV/AIDS and safer sex, Tina was unusual (in terms of our sample) in distinguishing between condom use and safer sex. She connected sexual safety to her positive expectations of sexual pleasure and her willingness to redefine 'normal' sexual conventions.

> *Q:* Did you change your behaviour? [because of HIV/AIDS]
> *T:* Yes I did, not in cutting down the relationships I've had. . . . What I did, I made sure I had sheaths and also safe sex.
> *Q:* What do you understand as safe sex?
> *T:* Safe sex is as pleasurable an experience as actual penetration. Oral sex, just things like touching somebody else's body in a very gentle way. Kissing. Appreciating one another's bodies.

I think it's as [much] fun, if not more. You concentrate on each other's needs a lot more, you're a lot more aware of them. You're aware of each other's bodies a lot more. . . . Instead of 20 minutes of bang, bang, bang, you've got a whole night; you watch the dawn come up and you're still there.

Q: Have you had to convert your partners? Have you come across men who understand sex as being more than penetration?

T: Yes . . . I've said 'I don't want to do that', or 'why don't you try this?' Before they know it they're converted, and they suddenly realize — 'well we haven't actually done it' — 'Well I'm tired now, haven't you had a good time?' You can change a lot of people's ideas.

Tina's account indicates something of the possibilities of intellectual/experiential empowerment, even though this is very far from the practice of most young women. The challenge to sex education is now to consider how such practices can be effectively promoted to more conventional young women. Educating young people in positive models of masculine and feminine sexuality, while also attempting to transform the model of male sexuality which informs young men's sexual practices, is a major social undertaking (Thomson and Scott, 1990a).

Conclusions

This small group of relatively empowered young women may not all have been successful in achieving safer sex, but they stand out from the rest of the sample in the extent to which they have reflected on their experience and thought critically about what they do and what has happened to them. This process of critical reflection seems to be an important factor in the struggle for experiential empowerment since effective strategies for safer sex for women necessarily confront the current dominance of men's needs in sexual relationships.

We cannot think of empowerment as achieving safer sex simply in terms of encouraging more assertive individuals. Empowerment has to be a collective project which shifts the balance of power between women and men throughout society. The examples we have picked out show something of the daunting obstacles which face assertive young women who try to put their intellectual empowerment into practice. These obstacles are rooted in women's own conceptions of masculinity and femininity as well as broader social pressures and in men's behaviour. Our five case studies illustrate the ambiguity concerning a women's rights over her own body within heterosexual sexual culture. However, it is these very issues — a woman's sense of ownership of her body, the independence of her sexuality — that are vital components of intellectual empowerment. If conventions of sexual practice which are 'safe' in the sense of pregnancy, STDs and HIV/AIDS are to be transformed, empowerment must be not only intellectual but also experiential. Intellectually it means women being able to challenge the status quo of heterosexual sexual interaction. In practice it entails personally and generally confronting men with the possibilities of a positive female sexuality.

We have conceived young women's empowerment in terms of their ability to change not only their sexual behaviour, but also men's behaviour towards them in developing strategies for safer sex (see Wellings, 1988). In the long term, safer sex must be a set of strategies which women can carry with them between relationships. If young women depend on non-penetrative sex, then they have a strategy which is difficult to achieve in practice, but is a form of safer sex which travels with the person rather than being dependent on the context of sexual encounters. Maintaining a sense of personal empowerment which is independent of context and relationship can be difficult and lonely. It requires young women to negotiate a new model of sexuality which treats female sexual pleasure as a priority, and it has not yet been taken seriously by the health education establishment.

Since the process of empowerment in the lives of young women constitutes a challenge to male power, being empowered does not mean that young women can provide themselves with total protection in every risky sexual situation. Safer sex for young women constitutes a challenge to the ideas, identities, expectations and practices of men. Empowerment remains a contested process, and we recognize the categories of empowerment that we have used as unstable categories. Intellectual/experiential empowerment, however, does mean the power to recognize the constraints of different sexual situations, to define women's needs and to negotiate choices within these constraints. When young women manage the negotiation of sexual encounters safely, it is because they are managing their own lives.

Notes

1 We have defined empowerment as ways in which, and routes through which, young women can attempt to, or do take control over their own sexual activity and/or relationships.

2 The Women, Risk and AIDS Project is staffed by the authors working collectively, and has been financed by a two-year grant from the Economic and Social Research Council. It has also received a small grant from Goldsmiths' College, University of London Research Fund. Valuable assistance has been given by Jane Preston, Polly Radcliffe and Janet Ransom. WRAP has used a purposive sample to interview 150 young women aged 16–21 in London and Manchester in depth, and has additional data from 500 questionnaires. The Leverhulme Trust has given a further one-year grant for a study of young men, and for comparison of the two studies.

3 The average age at first sexual intercourse of the twenty-two sexually active young women in the sub-set discussed in this chapter was 15.95 years. In the sample as a whole the average age was 15.4 years: for middle-class young women the average was 16.27 years; for working-class young women it was 14.49 years.

4 Analysis of the ways in which this sub-set of young women respond to male violence in sexual relationships, and how these responses may be related to empowerment, is dealt with in Holland *et al.* (1991b).

5 For discussion of the theory of rational choice see Hindess (1988). The use of this model in HIV/AIDS health promotion has been criticized by Watney (1990).

6 Kate and Rachel Thomson in discussion.

7 A systemic network is an analytic device suitable for the organization and categorization of qualitative data, preserving and representing some of the original essence

of these data. A network is an instrument for enabling theory to be tested, translating the language of, in this instance, the interview transcript into the language of the theory. This helps with the interpretation of the patterns and meanings in the data (Bliss *et al.*, 1983). The conceptual categories constituting the network can be derived exclusively from theoretical concepts, but in this case came from developing interaction between feminist and sociological theory, the responses of the subjects and the researchers' experiences of the interviews.

8 The network shown in Figure 1 is an attempt to draw a conceptual map of women's experiences of empowerment and disempowerment. We have tried too to indicate process in the network. The downward arrow indicates recursivity, in that the categories which follow are not mutually exclusive, and you can go into this part of the network as many times as it takes to categorize and decribe the datum, text or unit of experience adequately. The bracket indicates that the categories which follow should be co-selected. Individuals may, for example, be *experientially* or *intellectually* empowered, but it is most likely that there are elements of each. The concept of *experiential and intellectual* outlines possible directions and outcomes and should be used in relation to the *experiential* and *intellectual* categories.

9 For further discussion of methods see Thomson and Scott (1990) and Ramazanoglu (1990). WRAP working papers are available from the Tufnell Press (47 Dalmeny Road, London N7 ODY, Tel: 071 272 4861) at £3.00 each.

10 The names of the young women interviewed and of their partners have been changed to preserve confidentiality.

References

AZJEN, I. and FISHBEIN, M. (1980) *Understanding Attitudes and Predicting Social Behaviour*, New York, Prentice-Hall.

BUSS, J., MONK, M. and OGBORN, J. (eds) (1983) *Qualitative Data Analysis for Educational Research: a guide to the use of systemic networks*, London, Croom Helm.

CHRISTOPHERS, H. (1990) *AIDS Dialogue*, 8, pp. 5–7.

COWARD, R. (1987) 'Sex after AIDS', *The New Internationalist*, March.

ESTAUGH, V. and WHEATLEY, J. (1990) *Family Planning and Family Well-being*, London, Family Policy Studies Centre.

FREEMAN, R. and SCOTT, S. (1990) 'AIDS and prevention', Unpublished paper.

GROSS, A.E. and BELLEW-SMITH, M. (1983) 'A Social Psychological Approach to Reducing Pregnancy Risk in Adolescence', in D. BYRNE and W.A. FISHER (Eds), *Adolescence, Sex and Contraception*, New Jersey, Laurence Erlbaum Associates.

HANMER, J. and MAYNARD, M. (1987) *Women, Violence and Social Control*, London, Macmillan.

HANSON, S.L., MYERS, D.E. and GINSBURG, A.L. (1987) 'The Role of Responsibility and Knowledge in Reducing Out of Wedlock Childbearing', *Journal of Marriage and the Family*, 49, pp. 241–56.

HINDESS, B. (1988) *Choice, Rationality and Social Theory*, London, Unwin Hyman.

HOLLAND, J., RAMAZANOGLU, C., SCOTT, S., SHARPE, S. and THOMSON, R. (1991a) 'Between Embarrassment and Trust: Young Women and the Diversity of Condom Use', in P. AGGLETON, P. DAVIES and G. HART (Eds), *AIDS: Responses, Interventions and Care*, Lewes, Falmer Press.

HOLLAND, J., RAMAZANOGLU, C., SCOTT, S., SHARPE, S. and THOMSON, R. (1991b) 'Pressured Pleasure: Young Women and the Negotiation of Sexual Boundaries', Paper given to the Annual Conference of the British Sociological Association, Manchester.

HUNT, S.M. and MACLEOD, M. (1987) 'Health and Behavioural Change: Some Lay Perspectives', *Community Medicine*, 9, 1, pp. 68–76.

JESSOP, L. and THOROGOOD, N. (1989) 'The Sociology of a Sex Education Project', Paper presented to the British Sociological Association Annual Conference, Plymouth.

KELLY, L. (1988) *Surviving Sexual Violence*, Cambridge, Polity Press.

KENT, V., DAVIES, M., DEVERELL, K. and GOTTESMAN, S. (1990) 'Social Interaction Routines Involved in Heterosexual Encounters: Prelude to First Intercourse', Paper presented at the Fourth Social Aspects of AIDS Conference, South Bank Polytechnic, London.

OFFICE OF POPULATION CENSUSES AND SURVEYS (1991) *OPCS Monitor* PP2, 91/1, London, OPCS.

RAMAZANOGLU, C. (1990) *Methods of Working as a Research Team*, WRAP Paper 3, London, Tufnell Press.

RAVEN, B.H. and LITMAN-ADIZES, T. (1986) 'Interpersonal Influence and Social Power in Health Promotion', in T.Z. SALISBURY *et al.* (Eds), *Advances in Health Education and Promotion, Vol. 1*, London, JAI Press.

RUMBOLD, J. (1991) 'Goodbye to All That', *The Guardian*, 13 March.

SETTERS, J. (1988) 'Safer Sex Guidelines for Heterosexuals', *Health Education Journal*, 47, 3 and 4, pp. 61–2.

STANKO, E. (1985) *Intimate Intrusions: Women's Experience of Male Violence*, London, Routledge and Kegan Paul.

THOMSON, R. and SCOTT, S. (1990a) *Learning about Sex: Young Women and the Social Construction of Sexual Identity*, WRAP Paper 4, London, Tufnell Press.

THOMSON, R. and SCOTT, S. (1990b) *Researching Sexuality in the Light of AIDS: Historical and Methodological Issues*, WRAP Paper 5, London, Tufnell Press.

THOMPSON, S. (1984) 'Searching for Tomorrow: On Feminism and the Reconstruction of Teen Romance', in C. VANCE (Ed.), *Pleasure and Danger: Exploring Female Sexuality*, London, Routledge and Kegan Paul.

WATNEY, S. (1990) 'AIDS: The Second Decade: "Risk", Research and Modernity', in P. AGGLETON, P. DAVIES and G. HART (Eds), *AIDS: Responses, Interventions and Care*, Lewes, Falmer Press.

WELLINGS, K. (1988) 'Do We Need to Change Sexual Behaviour, Should We, Can We?' *Health Education Journal*, 47, 3 and 4, pp. 57–60.

WILLIAMS, D. (1990) Interview with Mukesh Kapila, *AIDS Dialogue*, 8, pp. 3–4.

WILTON, T. and AGGLETON, P.J. (1990) 'Condoms, Coercion and Control: AIDS and Heterosexual Practice', in P. AGGLETON, P. DAVIES and G. HART (Eds), *AIDS: Responses, Interventions and Care*, Lewes, Falmer Press.

12 The Limitations of Rational Decision-Making Models as Applied to Young People's Sexual Behaviour

Roger Ingham, Alison Woodcock and Karen Stenner

Much theorizing regarding health-related behaviours is based on an assumption of individual rationality. Probably the most widely used formal approach — the Health Belief Model — proposes that individuals arrive at health-relevant decisions after taking due account of a number of factors. These include the perceived severity of the condition, the level of risk, the costs and benefits of alternative behaviour changes, and the presence of cues to action (Maiman and Becker, 1974; Rosenstock, 1974). More recent versions have added or adapted variables; one such addition has been the concept of self-efficacy, or the extent to which individuals feel that they have control over the course of events (Rosenstock *et al.*, 1988).

A further widely used theoretical approach in social and health psychology refers to rationality in its very title — the Theory of *Reasoned* Action (Fishbein and Azjen, 1975; Azjen and Fishbein, 1980), and its successor, the Theory of *Planned* Behaviour (Azjen, 1988). These models propose that behavioural intentions are the best predictors of subsequent behaviour. Intentions, in turn, can be predicted by the beliefs and knowledge regarding the behaviour in question, together with the subjective norms. These relate to the extent to which individuals believe that important others would wish them to engage, or not as the case may be, in the particular behaviour(s). The relative influence of beliefs and subjective norms varies with different domains of behaviour.

These and similar models are referred to quite frequently in the HIV/AIDS literature in attempts to improve the prediction of behavioural outcomes (for example, Emmons *et al.*, 1986; McKusick *et al.*, 1985; Rutter, 1989). They also appear to guide the thinking behind much of the effort which goes into publicity campaigns, both national and local, in the field of HIV education. Thus, after the population had been made aware of the existence of HIV infection and its consequences, attention turned to specific pieces of advice intended to alter belief structures of individuals. For example, the Chief Medical Officer for England was widely quoted recently as saying, 'my advice to anyone who has vaginal intercourse with someone they do not know well is that they wear a condom or ensure one is worn. I am not aware of any better advice other than they do not have sex with someone they do not know' (*The Daily Telegraph*, 16 October 1990). More recent campaigns have stressed that HIV-associated risk is not restricted to certain 'types' of people, and so on.

At a more local level there is evidence that such approaches are prevalent in many school-based interventions. For example, Stears and Clift (1990), on the basis of their study of secondary schools in the South East Thames Region, report that 'information-giving' (as opposed to participative) approaches are adopted by the majority of teachers. Indeed, they report that such methods appear to increase in popularity as the age of the pupils increases. Similar results were obtained in a study of teachers in Hampshire schools and colleges. In response to items concerning how effective a number of different possible approaches were thought to be, the highest ratings were obtained for 'giving information', followed (in order) by 'calling in medical help', 'setting up a play', 'role plays about condoms' and 'trying to frighten' (Ingham and Henderyckx, in preparation). Such campaigns and interventions rest on the assumption that 'correcting' false beliefs and misconceptions (often in biomedical terms) will enable or encourage any 'rational' person to alter their behaviour in the 'desired' direction. There are, however, some fundamental errors in this approach.

The first is methodological: using formal models of this kind requires the use of questionnaires to enable the production of scores on the relevant dimensions. Quite apart from not insignificant problems of ensuring that the items are understood by all respondents in a similar manner (see, for example, Coxon, 1988), and that the response categories are unambiguous and appropriate, there are major difficulties in interpretation. For example, the probability that the same response to a particular item may be produced for a variety of different reasons is often overlooked, and the aggregated statistical relationships between variables are usually interpreted in simple explanatory modes. The range of possible explanations is limited by the variables incorporated in the model.

There is accumulating evidence that the Health Belief Model, for example, shows poor prediction of health-related behaviour in general (for example, Reid and Christensen, 1988; Rosenstock *et al.*, 1988) or of behavioural change in the HIV-related area (for example, Montgomery *et al.*, 1989; Hingson *et al.*, 1990; Fitzpatrick, Boulton and Hart, 1989; Brown *et al.*, in press).

The second major error is the assumption that the concept of 'rationality' is appropriate for the understanding of sexual behaviour. In other words, we are faced with evidence that young people appear (at least from superficial questionnaire data) to be very well informed regarding the major routes of HIV transmission, and yet do not appear to be adopting safer sexual practices on a wide scale (Ford and Bowie, 1989; Clift and Stears, 1989; Abrams *et al.*, 1990; Ingham, 1990). We are only surprised, or disturbed, by this apparent inconsistency to the extent that we have an implicit assumption that there should indeed be a rational link between these beliefs and the relevant behaviours.

Drawing on data from our own ESRC funded project on social aspects of risk reduction in young people, we have identified a number of impediments which forced us to challenge the notion of a direct and rational link between beliefs and behaviour. Many of these confirm, and in some cases elaborate, areas identified in other research projects, but are nevertheless worth reporting here in some detail. Our own study involves qualitative data collected from over 220 detailed interviews with young people aged between 16 and 25 years, concerning aspects of lifestyle, relationships and sexual histories, as well as matters concerning HIV-associated risk. The interviews were conducted by Alison Woodcock, Karen Stenner, Belinda Bateman and Jeremy Braybrooke and lasted between one and a half and three and a half hours. The vast majority of our respondents reported on exclusively heterosexual activities.

The seven impediments identified, which are not mutually exclusive, can be regarded both as impediments to our acceptance of the notion of rationality, and as impediments which intervene between what many young people 'know' and their willingness and/or ability to act on such 'knowledge'.

Perceived Invulnerability

Abrams and his colleagues (1990) have reported data from questionnaire surveys showing that young people are generally aware of the seriousness of HIV and the potential threat to others of their age group, and yet rate their own risk as very low. Memon (1991) has provided a review of some of the social psychological processes which may be involved, drawing attention to a range of attributional biases, as well as the need to locate the more individual cognitive approaches in a wider social context. Our own qualitative material has identified eighteen different reasons which help to maintain this perceived invulnerability (Woodcock *et al.*, 1992); these can be categorized under a number of headings. Some simply deny the risk, for example: 'I think its been blown up; I don't think its worth bothering about' (Female, 17). Other comments relate to perceptions of general risk. These include evidence of optimistic bias — 'It's never going to happen to me' — a greater fear of other problems, like pregnancy, a dismissal of the advice received since some of it is seen as impossible to put into practice — 'you can't go round not having sex, can you?', and a specific rejection of the risk of HIV on the grounds that life is full of so many risks that one in particular should not be given undue priority. An idiosyncratic observation is provided in this example:

> I can't go through life being scared of everything . . . I mean I could be run over by a bus . . . statistics I've read about AIDS . . . I've got more chance of being run over by a bus than dying of AIDS . . . so I think I should . . . I think if I got run over by a bus I would worry and think Jeez, I could get AIDS, but until a bus actually comes for me, I shan't bother, I don't think. . . . (Male, 20).

We accept that it can be argued that acknowledgment of the risk, coupled with a 'fatalistic' bias (that is, that chance factors are paramount), implies a different set of psychological processes from those involved in beliefs of personal invulnerability. We have included this 'belief' under this category, however, since, like the 'purer' forms of personal invulnerability, the perceived need for change is denied. Further exploration of the dynamics of these ways of understanding may well lead us to create a separate category.

A further category relates to perceptions of, and attributions about, partners. Those aspects of partners that are regarded as indicating 'safety' include their not being seen as 'promiscuous', that they are 'faithful', that they have had only 'serious' relationships previously, that they gave the 'impression' of being safe through their appearance, general personality, family and/or job, that they had been tested, that they were 'known' by the respondent (see below), and that if the partner had 'had AIDS they would have told me'. Thus, for example: 'You can usually tell — the lads are the ones that get AIDS . . . the lads that go round and do . . . screw anything in a skirt . . . you don't have to ask because you can tell by the way they come onto you' (Female, 17).

Finally, comments made about themselves by our respondents to indicate invulnerability include that they are 'not in a high risk group', that they are 'not promiscuous' nor 'go in for one-night stands', that they always use condoms when they think it is necessary, that they have been tested and that they do not have sex in high-risk areas, variously identified as London, USA, Spain and parts of Glasgow.

Feelings of invulnerability are enabled and maintained through a wide range of conceptions and misconceptions, in many cases indicating an understanding of particular parts of the 'received wisdom', and filling out the gaps with 'knowledge' gained from the media, from friends or from 'common sense'. Particularly false knowledge arose in some cases regarding the role of testing, in that some respondents reported that they (or their partners) had had blood tests for one condition and assumed that it would have been routinely tested for HIV (and that they would have been told had there been a problem).

Range of Understandings of Terminologies

Warwick *et al.*'s (1988) early work on the range of understandings regarding the specific nature of HIV infection demonstrated variation in the extent to which their young respondents felt that reduction of risk was (or was not) within their own control. Similar examples of a range of alternative meanings emerge from close examination of a number of concepts in our transcripts. We shall use one as an example: this concerns the phrase 'get to know your partner'. One of the major planks of the 'official' advice is 'use a condom if you don't know your partner.' Many of our respondents felt that they do indeed 'know' their partners so, as a matter of simple logic, they do not see the need for condom use. The issue is, however, whether their concept of 'knowing' coincides with that intended in the 'official' advice. It rarely does: superficial judgments based on having been acquainted with someone for some years, knowledge of the person's occupation, place of residence or parents' occupations are often regarded as sufficient criteria. Rarely was there any reported knowledge based on actual discussions regarding previous sexual activities, although in some cases reputations, based on rumour and gossip, figured prominently. For example,

> Wayne says 'she's alright, don't worry about it' and I might say to Clare, you know, 'what have you found her like, what's she like?', and she says 'don't worry, she's . . .', not in so many words but sometimes I get 'oh she's been going out with a boyfriend for a couple of months and she's a bit fed up now — yeah, she's gone out with one or two other blokes, but not many . . .' . . . mostly I would ask the lads what they think of them and they exaggerate and then after, I sort of like take everything with a pinch of salt. (Male, 16)

We have looked closely at the reports regarding knowledge of partner at first intercourse, and how this covaried with other aspects. Overall, one-third of respondents reported knowing absolutely nothing; a similar proportion reported *actual* knowledge of sexual status (that is, virgin or not), while a slightly lower proportion reported *assumed* knowledge. Just 16 per cent reported knowing some datails of their partner's sexual histories. Usually, this was only the number or 'seriousness' of previous relationships, not details of condom use or other specific details. Around a quarter of the females reported their first ever intercourse when they were 14 years or less; this often occurred very early in a relationship when they knew nothing at all about their partners, and condom use was rare (cf. Ingham *et al.*, 1991).

Positive Reasons for Non-Rationality

In many cases we found evidence that our respondents knew what was the 'appropriate' course of action but had developed positive reasons why such advice could, or should, not be followed. Again, we will use examples concerning revelations of prior sexual experience.

Reputational issues featured prominently. Some respondents felt that to report on previous activities could be seen as bragging (which, although acceptable in many male contexts, was not generally thought to be acceptable in the context of a relationship). At the other extreme, those with little or no experience reported embarrassment at the prospect of revealing this to actual or potential partners. Clearly, since self-disclosure generally operates in a reciprocal fashion, an unwillingness on the part of one partner to begin, or respond to, such discussions makes them rather short-lived.

Further reasons included possible effects on the relationship itself. Some respondents reported feelings of jealousy whenever reference was made to previous partners, as in the following example:

> ... in the early days I was concerned ... because I was too emotionally wrapped up in it all, so it would really hurt me to think about the guys that had been there before me. Now I don't bother because I'm a guy that has been there before somebody, you know. (Male, 25)

Others were quite clear in accepting that knowing too much about the other's past would constitute a 'turn-off'. For example:

> I don't think I know anybody that has sort of sat down and said 'what's your sexual background?' It's not a case of that ... it's really quite silly actually because you should ... 'how many girls have you slept with?' ... 'oh, can't count, can't remember' ... I think it's more that you don't want to know. You would think 'oh God, if they've slept with that many, oh, I don't want to sleep with them', so even though you want them, so you don't ask. If you ask, then you don't want them anymore, so you go home and then you think, 'wish I'd stayed now', you know. (Female, 17)

A further argument revolved around the assumption that a partner who revealed details of their own sexual history would, in due course, reveal details of their current activities to future partners. Thus potential 'victims' of such future exposure of intimate details tend to want to discourage such conversations. For example:

> Like I always say to him, 'if we finish, you better not tell anyone . . . you know, the things we have done and everything', and he always says 'oh, as if I would' he says 'do I say anything about, you know, other girls?' which is true. So I do trust him. I don't know, and I still don't feel real comfortable. (Female, 17)

It is important to understand from these brief examples that the explanations given are perfectly rational from within the framework of the respondents' own positions and/or understandings. Our intention is to point out the ways in which these various rationalities are at odds with, and counteract, the 'received rationality' of official biomedical wisdom.

External and Internal Pressures

Rational decision-making models assume a level of independent and free choice after weighing up the various pieces of information. The models do not generally account adequately for the powerful effects of pressures of various kinds. In keeping with other researchers (for example, Lees, 1986), we have found clear evidence of the effects of peer or media pressure to engage in intercourse, especially among males, but not uncommon in females. Again, reputational features are crucial in understanding the processes involved here; for roughly half of the males, to be sexually active was felt to be 'demanded' by peer groups. For females, although there were some for whom losing a reputation as a 'fridge' was very important, sexual experience outside a caring relationship was considered unacceptable in many contexts.

In some cases these external pressures become internalized, such that beliefs about what constitutes a 'real' man or woman provided strong pressures to become sexually active, even though there was no immediate intention of telling others about it. The notion of reputation can be applied equally with regard to 'self as audience' as to 'other as audience'.

Other forms of external pressures included force, either physical or emotional, and, not surprisingly, women were considerably more likely to be the victims. When reporting how they felt about their first ever intercourse after the event, many women reported strong feelings of regret and self-recrimination. For example:

> . . . [there was no pleasure] . . . because all I could think about was how much pain I was going through at the time and I couldn't really settle down and enjoy it because it was just hurting me too much . . . but even though he said he was trying to do it as gently as possible — to prevent me from being hurt — I was still hurt . . . and afterwards I just felt used and cheated by it all and I still went ahead and done it again . . . [*AW*: why did you feel used and cheated?] . . . because I didn't love him and I knew

he didn't love me, and I didn't really feel anything for him and didn't expect anything to happen . . . whether he did or not I don't know, but because I didn't love him . . . and I always believed that it would be someone I loved first and it wasn't so I felt a bit out of order for that, so I cheated myself more than anything, nobody else (Female, 16)

The very few men who experienced regret had had their first ever experience with older women.

The approximately one-quarter of respondents who referred to being 'carried away' included many who had an awareness of what they *should* (or should not) do, but claimed that they felt unable to control themselves. For example:

I regretted it, I really did. I thought 'oh God, this is not the way to lose it' . . . you are supposed to lose it in a meaningful relationship, you know. You're supposed to do it after you've known a guy for five months, six months, you know. There's me on my one night stand, pissed as hell, and lose it in someone else's bedroom, you know. I thought, 'great, well done'. (Female, 17)

I wasn't drunk. I can remember everything I was doing, but if I hadn't been drinking I wouldn't have done everything I did do. (Female, 17)

Ideologies and Power

Findings from the Women, Risk and AIDS Project identify the importance of gender ideologies as factors influencing women's and men's sexual behaviour (Holland *et al.*, 1990, 1991). Similarly, the different discourses highlighted by authors such as Hollway (1984) are valuable in making sense of our data. Analysis of the various ways in which respondents related to such discourses suggests that some respondents appeared to accept certain positions unquestioningly, while others purposely rejected certain positions by making reference to the fact that they 'were not like the others, who. . . .' The limited extent to which such discourses are available for subjective analysis poses a serious challenge to the concepts of rationality and individual decision-making contained in the models of health behaviour mentioned earlier.

The Mystique of Sexual Behaviour

Different social constructions of sexual activity emerge from our transcripts; some are based on moral conceptions, and some on the notion of natural and spontaneous behaviour. The majority contain a central essence involving mystique. Many respondents referred to the avoidance of the topic by parents, the embarrassment of many teachers to go beyond the biological, and the ways in which coy language and *double entendres* are used in the media, by adults and within relationships. This construction of sexual activity as something mystical is hardly an adequate preparation for considered thinking, however defined.

This social construction makes it very difficult for prospective sexual partners to talk to each other in specific terms about activities, more generally relying on vague and evasive phrases (such as 'doing it', 'being careful', 'using something' and so on). It also 'gives permission' to people to behave in certain ways. 'I don't know what came over me' or 'I'm not usually like that' are common and acceptable justifications for what might appear to themselves and others to be 'aberrant' behaviour. In other words, the examples cited earlier, in which people were clearly aware of the discrepancy between what they *should* do and what they *did* do, can be internally justified and accepted, since the construction of sexual activity involves assumptions of mystical and uncontrollable forces.

It is in consideration of this topic that we can begin to map out a possible role for the concept of 'rationality'. Rather than regarding it as an inherent 'property' of individuals (as implied by some of the psychological models), or as an overwhelming force, we should regard it as an option. In other words, people can *choose* on what basis they will make decisions — always subject to (often powerful) constraints. It is an option to be considered alongside other options, subject to the proviso that we may be (and often are) called to account for our behaviour (cf. Harre, 1979). The social contexts in which such accounting, or warranting, takes place, as well as the nature of what is being accounted for, determine the extent to which 'rationality' is an acceptable justification for actions both for others-as-audience and for selves-as-audience.[1]

Regarding rationality as an option has implications for the way we regard the concepts of 'costs' and 'benefits', as used, for example, in the Health Belief Model (HBM) (Ingham, 1992). Rather than basing these in terms of *specific* biomedical and health-preserving actions or behaviours (common in many applications of the HBM), we should afford greater priority to the importance of reputations and identities within particular social worlds.

Negotiation and Joint Decision-Making

The final impediment to the acceptance of a notion of rational and individual decision-making models as applied to sexual activity is the obvious point that it is a joint effort. From our data it is clear that 'negotiation' regarding safer sexual practices, such as it is, tends to be based on assertion and insistence, and was almost inevitably concerned with avoidance of conception rather than with avoidance of infection.[2] For example, one young man told us: 'She produced condoms from the glove compartment of her car . . . She just said "Do you know what these are for?' . . . I said "yes" . . . and she said "good — use it" . . . so I thought, "right, fair enough"' (Male, 17).

In many cases, however, responsibility was assumed, and little was said. Among the potentially important factors here are the clash of different lay beliefs, the use of threats, power differentials in terms of gender, age or experience, and the use and effectiveness of warranting statements, justifications. Some of these aspects will be explored when we analyze the results of a hypothetical role-play study in which individuals were confronted with various situations and asked to report how they thought they could (and would) respond. Through this approach we will be able to explore the resources available for negotiation, and some of the reasons why, in practice, these resources do not appear to be fully utilized.

Discussion

The notion of a direct link between beliefs and behaviour is simply not tenable. In the cases of some of the impediments identified, it may be reasonable to think in terms of a range of 'rationalities', depending on the identities and social worlds of the individuals concerned (a similar point has been argued by Prieur, 1990a, 1990b). In other cases, people are aware of what is acknowledged to be the 'rational' response, but are unable to adhere to it. In still further cases, the very notion that people have any awareness of, or control over, their behaviour must be challenged. Lest we give the impression that we are implying that young people are unique in these regards, we are sure that detailed consideration of the sexual behaviour of many adults would reveal a similar picture.

This analysis also has implications for health promotion. Simple unidirectional messages will be relatively ineffective since they cannot hope to address the many and varied positions with which they are confronted. The millions of pounds spent on national media campaigns could alternatively create a large number of jobs to provide the opportunity for intensive and interactive work in small group settings. Some of the impediments identified might well require long-term social transformation (cf. Homans and Aggleton, 1988), but others can be addressed in the meantime.

New theoretical approaches to understanding health-related behaviour require a shift away from an obsession with individual knowledge or attitude scores on questionnaires towards the elucidation of meanings, powers, liabilities and constraints, from simple concepts of illness avoidance towards an acknowledgment of the importance of social reputations, and from crude frequencies towards the dynamic processes involved in creating and maintaining identities. Although new and improved modelling is essential, we are doubtful whether the traditional reliance on individual scores and the production of statistical linkages between the components of such models will lead to the level of understanding required.

Finally, other than referring to the use of the concept in health behaviour models, we have failed to attempt any definition of the term 'rational'. *Chambers Twentieth Century Dictionary* (1952 edition) provides a definition which only serves to confirm the problematic issue of who is to be the arbiter of what is, or is not, 'rational'.

> *rational, adj.* of the reason: endowed with reason: agreeable to reason: sane: intelligent: judicious: commensurable with natural numbers. — *noun* a rational being or quantity: (in *plural*) rational dress, i.e., knickerbockers instead of skirt.

Notes

1 Gold (1989) offers a revealing account of some of the justifications produced for self and others in the context of safe and unsafe sex among gay men.
2 Although, of course, the former is a more likely outcome, the point is that very few respondents commented on the dual functions of condoms in risk reduction.

References

ABRAMS, D., ABRAHAM, C., SPEARS, R. and MARKS, D. (1990) 'AIDS Invulnerability: Relationships, Sexual Behaviour and Attitudes among 16 to 19 year olds', in P. AGGLETON, P. DAVIES and G. HART (Eds), *AIDS: Individual, Cultural and Policy Dimensions*, Lewes, Falmer Press.

AZJEN, I. (1988) *Attitudes, Personality and Behaviour*, Milton Keynes, Open University Press.

AZJEN, I. and FISHBEIN, M. (1980) *Understanding Attitudes and Predicting Social Behaviour*, Englewood Cliffs, N.J., Prentice-Hall.

BROWN, L.K., DICLEMENTE, R.J. and REYNOLDS, L.A. (in press) 'HIV Prevention for Adolescents: Utility of the Health Belief Model', *AIDS Education and Prevention*.

CLIFT, S. and STEARS, D. (1989) 'Undergraduates' Beliefs and Attitudes about AIDS', in P. AGGLETON, P. DAVIES and G. HART (Eds), *AIDS: Social Representations and Social Practices*, Lewes, Falmer Press.

COXON, A. (1988) 'The Numbers Game: Gay Lifestyles, Epidemiology of AIDS and Social Science', in P. AGGLETON and H. HOMANS (Eds), *Social Aspects of AIDS*, Lewes, Falmer Press.

EMMONS, C.A., JOSEPH, J.G., Kessler, R.C., WORTMAN, C.B., MONTGOMERY, S.B. and OSTROW, D.G. (1986) 'Psychosocial Predictors of Reported Behavior Change in Homosexual Men at Risk for AIDS', *Health Education Quarterly*, 13, pp. 331–45.

FISHBEIN, M. and AZJEN, I. (1975) *Belief, Attitude, Intention and Behaviour: An Introduction to Theory and Research*, Reading, Mass., Addison-Wesley.

FITZPATRICK, R. BOULTON, M. and HART, G. (1989) 'Gay Men's Sexual Behaviour in Response to AIDS: Insights and Problems', in P. AGGLETON, G. HART and P. DAVIES (Eds), *AIDS: Social Representations, Social Practices*, Lewes, Falmer Press.

FORD, N. and BOWIE, C. (1989) 'Urban-Rural Variations in the Level of Heterosexual Activity of Young People', *Area*, 21, 3, pp. 237–48.

GOLD, R. (1989) 'Situational Factors and Thought Processes Associated with Unprotected Sexual Intercourse in Gay Men', Unpublished paper, School of Education, Deakin University, Victoria 3217, Australia.

HARRE, R. (1979) *Social Being: A Theory for Social Psychology*, Oxford, Basil Blackwell.

HINGSON, R.W., STRUNIN, L., BERLIN, B.M. and HEEREN, T. (1990) 'Beliefs about AIDS, Use of Alcohol and Drugs, and Unprotected Sex among Massachusetts Adolescents', *American Journal of Public Health*, 80, pp. 295–9.

HOLLAND, J., RAMAZANOGLU, C. and SCOTT, S. (1990a) 'Managing Risk and Experiencing Danger: Tensions between Government AIDS Education Policy and Young Women's Sexuality', *Gender and Education*, 2, 2, pp. 125–46.

HOLLAND, J., RAMAZANOGLU, C., SCOTT, S., SHARP, S. and THOMSON, R. (1991) 'Between Embarrassment and Trust: Young Women and the Diversity of Condom Use', in P. AGGLETON, P. DAVIES and G. HART (Eds), *AIDS: Responses, Interventions and Care*, Lewes, Falmer Press.

HOLLWAY, W. (1984) 'Gender Differences and the Production of Subjectivity', in J. HENRIQUES, W. HOLLWAY, C. URWIN, V. COUZE and V. WALKERDINE, *Changing the Subject: Psychology, Social Regulation and Subjectivity*, London, Methuen.

HOMANS, H. and AGGLETON, P. (1988) 'Health Education, HIV Infection and AIDS', in P. AGGLETON and H. HOMANS (Eds), *Social Aspects of AIDS*, Lewes, Falmer Press.

INGHAM, R. (1990) 'Report of the Pre-Testing of the World Health Organisation's Young People's KABP Questionnaire', Unpublished report to WHO, University of Southampton.

INGHAM, R. (1992) 'Sexuality and Health in Young People', in G.N. PENNY, P. BENNETT and M. HERBERT (Eds), *Health Psychology: A Lifespan Perspective*, London, Harwood Academic Publishers.

INGHAM, R. and HENDERYCKX, A. (in preparation) 'Teachers' Views on Interventions Regarding HIV Infection', Department of Psychology, University of Southampton.

INGHAM, R., WOODCOCK, A. and STENNER, K. (1991) 'Getting to Know You . . . Young People's Knowledge of Their Partners at First Intercourse, *Journal of Community and Applied Social Psychology* (in press).

LEES, S. (1986) *Losing Out: Sexuality and Adolescent Girls*, London, Hutchinson.

MCKUSICK, L., WILEY, J., COATES, T.J., STALL, R., SAIKA, G., MORIN, S., CHARLES, K., HORSTMAN, W. and CONANT, M.A. (1985) 'Reported Changes in the Sexual Behaviour of Gay Men at Risk for AIDS, San Francisco 1982–1984: The AIDS Behavioral Research Project', *Public Health Reports*, 100, pp. 622–9.

MAIMAN, L.A. and BECKER, M.H. (1974) 'The Health Belief Model: Origins and Correlates in Psychological Theory', in M.H. BECKER (Ed.), *The Health Belief Model and Personal Health Behaviour*, Thorofare, N.J., Charles B. Slack.

MEMON, A. (1991) 'Perceptions of AIDS Vulnerability: The Role of Attributions and Social Context', in P. AGGLETON, P. DAVIES and G. HART (Eds), *AIDS: Responses, Interventions and Care*, Lewes, Falmer Press.

MONTGOMERY, S.B., JOSEPH, J.G., BECKER, M.H., OSTROW, D.G., KESSLER, R.C. and KIRSCHT, J.P. (1989) 'The Health Belief Model in Understanding Compliance with Preventative Recommendations for AIDS: How Useful?', *AIDS Education and Prevention*, 1, pp. 303–23.

PRIEUR, A. (1990a) 'Taking Risks Is Rational Behaviour: Experiences from the Use of Qualitative Research Methods'. Paper presented at the International Conference on Assessing AIDS Prevention, Montreux, 29 October to 1 November 1990.

PRIEUR, A. (1990b) 'Norwegian Gay Men: Reasons for Continued Practice of Unsafe Sex', *AIDS Education and Prevention*, 2, 2, pp. 109–15.

REID, L.D. and CHRISTENSEN, D.B. (1988) 'A Psychosocial Perspective in the Explanation of Patients' Drug-taking Behaviour', *Social Science and Medicine*, 27, pp. 277–85.

ROSENSTOCK, I.M. (1974) 'Historical Origins of the Health Belief Model', *Health Education Monographs*, 2, pp. 328–35.

ROSENSTOCK, I.M., STRECHER, V.J. and BECKER, M.H. (1988) 'Social Learning Theory and the Health Belief Model', *Health Education Quarterly*, 15, pp. 175–83.

RUTTER, D. (1989) 'Models of Belief-Behaviour Relationships in Health', *Health Psychology Update*, 4, pp. 3–10.

STEARS, D. and CLIFT, S. (1990) *A Survey of AIDS Education in Secondary Schools*, Horsham, AVERT.

WARWICK, I., AGGLETON, P. and HOMANS, H. (1988) 'Young People's Health Beliefs and AIDS', in P. AGGLETON and H. HOMANS (Eds), *Social Aspects of AIDS*, Lewes, Falmer Press.

WOODCOCK, A.J., STENNER, K. and INGHAM, R. (1992) 'Young People Talking about HIV and AIDS: Interpretations of Personal Risk of Infection', *Health Education Research; Theory and Practice* (in press).

13 'Obviously the Advice Is Then to Keep to Safer Sex': Advice-giving and Advice reception in AIDS Counselling

David Silverman, Robert Bor, Riva Miller and Eleanor Goldman

Amidst the polemics of what Watney (1987) has called 'AIDS commentary', there is general agreement about three issues: first, that 'AIDS is primarily a *social* phenomenon with urgent and consuming medical issues attached' (Miller, 1988, p. 130); second, that, short of a medical breakthrough, the most effective response to HIV infection is via cultural and behavioural change; and third, that such change will depend upon communication processes that are complicated and little understood.

While there is some support for health promotion programmes based simply on information (WHO, 1988, p. 15), most researchers and community workers argue that knowledge itself does not change behaviour (Stoller and Rutherford, 1989; Nelkin, 1987; Aggleton, 1989; Greenblat *et al.*, 1989) and that fear arousal is largely ineffective (Sherr, 1989). However, it remains difficult to isolate those factors which are effective in changing people's behaviour. For instance, a recent review of studies of the impact of HIV testing on behaviour reveals great uncertainties about the salient factors — is it testing, learning the result of one's test, or testing with counselling that is most effective in behaviour change (Miller and Pinching, 1989)?

It seems that the answer we give to these questions depends upon which wave of the epidemic we are talking about. Early research had suggested the effectiveness of a positive test result in producing behaviour change among gay men (Miller *et al.*, 1986; Peterman and Curran, 1986; Richards, 1986). However, this may have had a lot to do with the effective role of peer-endorsed safer sex ethics among the gay community. Testing alone is unlikely to be as effective with injecting drug users and heterosexuals facing the next wave of the epidemic (Miller and Pinching, 1989).

Where people lack a supportive peer network, HIV counselling has increasingly been proposed as 'a key component of programmes . . . both complementing and supporting information, education and communication strategies, and as a *sine qua non* of clinical management' (Carballo and Miller, 1989, p. 117). So it is argued, particularly in Britain, that there is a need to counsel all patients at STD clinics about HIV (Quinn, 1988) and that, in any event, counselling must precede the antibody test (Miller *et al.*, 1986). It is suggested that this is a matter not just of health education but also of social support — cases of suicide have been reported among people who have the HIV test without pre-counselling (Miller, 1988).

At whatever stage counselling takes place, attention must be paid to its form as well as its content. Some normative definitions take account of the social relationship between counsellor and client. For instance, Miller and Pinching (1989, p. 191) argue that: 'the counsellor in HIV must remain a person offering a trusting, implicitly and explicitly supportive, ongoing and confidential relationship that rises above the rhetoric, the hype, the unrealistic expectations and the hidden agendas embraced by . . . public discussions.' However, while few counsellors would disagree with this statement, it is not immediately clear how it could be carried out in practice or what are the mechanics through which such a 'trusting' relationship could produce a communication format able to generate client uptake a changed behaviour.

Reading the available literature, one is struck by the prevalence of well-meaning advice based on commonsense, liberal assumptions rather than on research. Fenton's (1987) emphasis on 'feeling comfortable' when discussing sex and on the counsellor knowing the right information is a case in point. Miller and Bor's (1988) discussion of different ways in which counsellors can construct questions is a rare exception to a literature which largely confines itself to generalities.

Two further factors, discussed in many reports, make this situation particularly worrying. First, large numbers of references are made to the current practical problems of HIV counselling — from staff 'burnout' (Carballo and Miller, 1989), to the pressures produced by media campaigns (Thompson and McIver, 1988; Beck *et al.*, 1987; Sonnex *et al.*, 1987) and the related problem of counselling an increasing group of 'worried well' (Miller, 1987; Salt *et al.*, 1989). Second, the training needs of groups as diverse as health advisors (Sadler, 1988) and social workers (Shernoff, 1988), as well as general practitioners and those working in primary care (Henry, 1988; Goedert, 1987; Hodgkin, 1988), seem immense and largely unsatisfied.

The lack of a soundly-based counselling practice is acknowledged in some of the literature. For instance, Carballo and Miller recognize that, despite normative definitions, what counts as counselling remains problematic. As they suggest, the ad hoc character of counselling practice is a common feature of examples elsewhere of crisis intervention:

> As a result, counselling strategies have often had to be innovative and hastily derived and, to date, much of the HIV/AIDS counselling support being provided continues to be the result of the personal commitment and interests of individual clinicians and other health care staff. As such, its characterisation, definition, role and content is variable and lacking in training support and institutionalised continuity. (Carballo and Miller, 1989, p. 119)

This chapter reports comparative material based on an intensive study of recordings of counselling in ten different centres in England, the USA and Trinidad. It deals with a small aspect of a larger research project (see also Perakyla and Bor, 1990; Silverman, 1990; Silverman and Perakyla, 1990; Silverman and Bor, 1991; Perakyla and Silverman, 1991a, 1991b).

Over 100 recordings from seven English clinics, and from two US and one Trinidad centres have been transcribed and analyzed. Video-recordings have also been obtained from the video archive of the Royal Free Hospital's Haemophilia Centre and District AIDS Unit, where extracts from thirty consultations have been transcribed and analyzed. Recording was based on the informed consent of patients on the understanding that their anonymity would be preserved. In this chapter we analyze audio transcripts.[1] Henceforth, we use P to refer to patients and C to counsellors. A complete set of transcription symbols is provided in an appendix to the chapter.

Why Advice?

Analyzing how advice is given and received was interesting for at least three reasons. First, the organization and reception of advice was identified as an issue important to one of our funding bodies, the Health Education Authority. If we could identity effective forms of advice-giving, then we would be fulfilling our mandate through making a direct contribution to the understanding of health promotion in face-to-face communication.

Second, earlier work had identified phenomena which provided an important context for the analysis of advice sequences. Initially, we had shown how counsellors and patients marked and managed the 'delicate' issues that arise in HIV/AIDS counselling like sexuality (Silverman and Perakyla, 1990; Silverman and Bor, 1991) and death (Perakyla and Bor, 1990). Clearly, the nature of such delicate topics would be likely to make advice-giving and reception particularly problematic.

Our subsequent work on the overall structure of communication between counsellors and patients (Perakyla and Silverman, 1991a) demonstrated that HIV counsellors use one of two kinds of communication formats as their 'home base': an Interview Format (in which Cs asks questions and Ps give answers) and an Information-Delivery Format (in which Cs deliver information and Ps are silent apart from small acknowledgment tokens). Other forms of communication (for instance, Ps asking questions or delivering information) turned out to be less common and more unstable. As we shall see, the research reported here has shown that advice-giving is also an unstable format. This has important implications both for our analysis and for its import for practice.

The third reason for focusing on advice was the fortuitous appearance of Heritage and Sefi's (forthcoming) work on the delivery and reception of advice in interactions between health visitors and first-time mothers. Although, as we show below, the different contexts (clinic versus home) and topics (sexuality and/or death versus babycare) of the two studies were to prove important, Heritage and Sefi gave us many of the analytic tools that were to be crucial in our analysis. It is thus important to offer a brief summary of their research.

Heritage and Sefi found that most advice sequences were initiated by the professional without any prior enquiry by the client. Health Visitor (HV)-initiated advice took four forms:

1 stepwise entry in the sequence below:

    a HV enquiry;
    b problem indicative response by client;

c request for specification by HV ('a focusing enquiry');
d a specification by the client;
e advice-giving;

2 the same sequence but with no request for specification because the client volunteers how she dealt with the problem;
3 no client statement of how she dealt with the problem and no HV request for specification (thus stages c and d are omitted);
4 HV-initiated advice without the client giving a problem indicative response (i.e., stage a is followed directly by stage e).

The majority of advice initiations analyzed were of Form 4. Indeed, in many cases even the HV's enquiry was not problem-oriented but was more concerned to topicalize the issue for which advice was subsequently delivered.

The reception of advice by mothers took three forms. In the first of these there was a marked acknowledgment (e.g., 'oh right' or repeats of key components of the advice); Heritage and Sefi say such utterances acknowledge the informativeness and appropriateness of the advice. In the second form there is an unmarked acknowledgment (e.g., 'mm', 'yeah', 'right' — without an 'oh'). These are minimal response tokens which have a primarily continuative function; they do *not* acknowledge the advice-giving as newsworthy to the recipient or constitute an undertaking to follow the advice, and can be heard as a form of resistance in themselves because, implicitly, such responses are refusing to treat the talk as advice. Third, there are assertions of knowledge or competence by the mother. These indicate that the advice is redundant — hence they also may be taken as resistance.

Heritage and Sefi's study shows that mothers minimize the extent to which they acknowledge that the advice of Health Visitors has been 'informative' (e.g., they found only one example of a 'newsworthiness' token — 'Oh'). Mothers rarely acknowledge their previous ignorance; nor do they receipt the HVs' talk as advice. Overwhelmingly, their most frequent response is an 'unmarked acknowledgment' via response tokens ('mm hm', 'yes', 'that's right') which do not constitute an undertaking to follow the advice offered.

However, where HVs used a step-wise entry into advice-giving (Form 1 above), they encountered less resistance and more uptake, displayed by mothers' use of marked acknowledgments. Here the HV's request for her client to specify a problem means that the advice can be recipient-designed, non-adversarial and not attribute blame. When discussed in this way, 'the potential need for advice can emerge as the joint construction of the participants' (Heritage and Sefi, forthcoming).

Advice: The AIDS Counselling Study

In our study the majority of advice sequences are initiated by the professional without the client giving a problem indicative response. Of the sixty-one advice sequences from five centres so far analyzed, a majority take Form 4 where the professional gives advice without any attempt to get the client to specify a problem. This is shown in Table 1.

Similarly, C-initiated advice appears to get little uptake (largely unmarked acknowledgments — henceforth UAs); conversely, full sequences get marked

Table 1 Forms of Advice-giving in HIV Counselling Data

Patient-initiated	2	
Counsellor-initiated	59	
Of which:	16	full sequence (Form 1)
	8	shortened sequence (Forms 2 and 3)
	35	C-initiated without problem-indicative response from P

Table 2 Form of Advice and Degree of Uptake

| Advice format | Number | Type of acknowledgment* | |
		unmarked	marked
P-initiated	2	0	2
C-initiated			
Step by step:			
full-sequence	11	1	10
Shortened	5	3	2
Truncated:			
no P problem elicited	32	29	3

Notes: Based on fifty advice sequences.
* 'Unmarked' means only unmarked acknowledgments were given in the advice sequence; 'marked' means that at least one marked acknowledgment was given.

acknowledgments (MAs). Predictably, the only example of a receipt of news token ('is that right', 'really') occurs when C has twice corrected a patient's statement. As in Heritage and Sefi's study, there is, however, little *overt* resistance to advice. The most common pattern is counsellor-initiated advice (not based on eliciting a perceived problem from the patient) interspersed with a series of 'mms'. The data on uptake are shown in Table 2.

Table 2 shows a clear correlation between the way in which an advice sequence is set up and the response it elicits from the patient. In the total of thirty-two cases where the counsellor delivers advice without attempting to generate a perceived problem from the patient, there are only three cases where the patient shows any sign of uptake. Conversely, in the other eighteen cases, where the advice emerges either at the request of the patient or in a step-by-step sequence, there are only four cases where the patient does *not* show uptake.

However, two further points need to be made about Table 2. First, we have deliberately excluded one centre from the analysis where we have examined eleven advice sequences. Here, although there are several examples of step-by-step advice packages, we find no marked acknowledgments and considerable overt resistance to advice. There is no space to look in detail at one of these deviant cases. It turns out that such advice packages do not get their predicted uptake because, although the advice follows a sequence of requests for specification, its content often does not take up or even contradicts the perceptions of the patient's problems that have been elicited. We have excluded these cases from Table 2 in order to show the more common pattern where advice sequences which follow step-by-step methods are constructed in terms of what the patient has just said.

The second point is that even within the fifty cases used here there are some unexpected examples. For instance, why should three examples of counsellor-initiated advice get marked acknowledgments, against the normal pattern? As Mitchell (1983) has forcefully argued, in case study work we have an obligation to follow up all deviant cases in order to strengthen the explanatory power of our analysis. Consequently, in Extract 3 below we examine one case of this kind. As it turns out, the analysis of this extract leads to an important conclusion about the advantages to the *counsellor* of giving advice without first eliciting a client's concerns.

How, then, do our data differ from those of Heritage and Sefi? First, we have comparative material available from several centres. We find that counsellors at any one centre tend to construct their advice packages in a similar manner. This offers a useful opportunity to test hypotheses and to highlight the consequences of different ways of giving advice.

Second, we have fewer cases of patient-initiated advice and fewer displays of patient competence. We can speculate that the different context is important here. A hospital interview about HIV may discourage displays of competence or knowledge by patients. To talk about looking after one's own baby in one's own home is one thing; to discuss a sexually transmitted disease is quite another. As our earlier research showed, patients only go into detail on potentially delicate topics, like sexuality, when specifically requested to do so by a professional (Silverman and Bor, 1991).

Third, unlike Heritage and Sefi, in addition to our main sample (sixty-one cases), we have seven further cases (from only two of five centres) where, although no advice is given by a counsellor, patients summarize what they have learned from the line of questioning. In Extract 6 below we examine how one patient can produce a version of what she has learned without any explicit advice sequence. As we argue, this has clear practice implications.

So far we have been talking in generalities. We now, therefore, examine our data, beginning with examples of the two main types of advice package: counsellor-initiated advice and a step-by-step sequence.

Extract 1

Counsellor-Initiated Advice

SW2-A
```
1   C:  .hhhh Now when someo:ne er is tested (.) and they
2       ha:ve a negative test result .hh it's obviously
3       dealuh:m that (.) they then look after themselves to
4       prevent [any further risk of=
5   P:          [Mm hm
6   C:  =infection. .hhhh I mean obviously this is only
7       possible up to a point because if .hhh you get into
8       a sort of serious relationship with someone that's
9       long ter:m .hh you can't obviously continue to use
10      condoms forever. .hh Uh:m and a point has to come
11      where you make a sort of decision (0.4) uh:m if you
12      are settling down about families and things that you
13      know (0.6) you'd- not to continue safer sex.
14      [.hhhh Uh:m but obviously: (1.0) you=
15  P:  [Mm:
```

```
16   C:   = nee:d to be (.) uh:m (.) take precautions uhm (0.3)
17        and keep to the safer practices .hhh if: obviously
18        you want to prevent infection in the future.
19   P:   [Mm hm
20   C:   [.hhhh The problem at the moment is we've got it
21        here in {names City} in particular (.) right across
22        the boar:d you know from all walks of life.
23   P:   Mm hm
24   C:   Uh::m from you know (.) the sort of established high
25        r- risk groups (.) now we're getting heterosexual
26        (.) [transmission as well. .hh Uhm=
27   P:       [Mm hm
28   C:   =so obviously everyone really needs to careful. .hhh
29        Now whe- when someone gets a positive test result
30        er: then obviously they're going to ke- think very
31        carefully about things. .hhh Being HIV positive
32        doesn't necessarily mean that that person is going
33        to develop ai:ds (.) later on.
34        (.)
35   P:   Mm hm
```

We can make four observations about this extract. First, C delivers advice without having elicited from P a perceived problem. Reasons of space do not allow us to include what immediately precedes this extract but it involves another topic (the meaning of a positive test result) and no attempt is made to question P about her possible response to this topic, that is, about how she might change her behaviour after a negative test result. Moreover, within this extract C introduces fresh topics (what to do in a 'serious' relationship on lines 6–13; the spread of HIV in the city on lines 20–22) without employing any 'step-by-step' approach. Second, predictably, the P only produces UAs (variations on 'mm hmm'). While these may indicate that P is listening, they do not mark what C is saying as advice. Hence, at the very least, they do not show P uptake and may also be taken as a sign of passive resistance. Third, there is no *active* resistance from P. Indeed, topic follows topic with a remarkable degree of smoothness and at great speed. Finally, C does not personalize her advice. Instead of using a personal pronoun or the patient's name, she refers to 'someone' and 'they' (lines 1–4) and 'everyone' (line 28).

Advice sequences like these are very common at three of the five centres examined. So we have to ask ourselves why counsellors should use a format which is likely to generate so little patient uptake. Since our preference is not to criticize professionals but to understand the logic of their work, we need to look at the *functions* as well as the dysfunctions of this way of proceeding. We do this later with reference to Extract 3.

Extract 2

Step-by-Step Advice

SS-2-16.1A

```
1   C:   Mm hm .hhh What sort of sexual relationship are you
2        having at the moment with him.
3        (0.6)
```

```
 4  P:   With X.
 5  C:   Mm hm
 6  P:   er::: (1.7) We:ll (0.6) hhhh God how to go into this
 7       on camera: I don't know. .hhhh er:: (2.6) Let me
 8       just say I'm on bottom he's on to:p, (0.7) er::
 9       There was a period at the very beginni:ng (0.5) er::
10       (0.5) where a condom was not- ((Clears throat))
11       excuse me was not used. (0.6)
12       er:[::
13  C:      [Are you using condoms now?=[Or er-
14  P:                                  [uh We::ll (0.4)
15       yeah. Mm (1.0) er::: (.) There is: (.) still some
16       oral se:x, (0.6) er:: not passing any fluids alo:ng
17       but they say: (0.4) that yes you do pass fluid
18       along. (0.4) So I'm still kind of nervous about
19       that.=However: .hhhh (0.2) er:uh::hhh (0.8) I:- I
20       don't know:: (0.5) what I don't know .hh is er::
21       (0.2) how: I would have contracted it to him.
22  C:   Mm:=
23  P:   =er::: (0.7) I have not (1.1) er:: (1.0) had anal
24       intercourse with hi:m.
25       (0.8)
26  C:   Okay.
27  P:   er::: (0.5) He ha:s
28  C:   Mm
29  P:   er:: (0.5) performed oral sex on me:
30       (.)
31  C:   M[m:
32  P:    [without a condo:m, (.) but I've not ejaculated
33       into his mouth.
34  C:   Mm
35  P:   er:: But (.) like they say you do (.) (lose some
36       though).
37  C:   Mm
38       (.)
39  P:   er::
40       (.)
41  C:   Yeah. .h I think (.) Paul how we understand things
42       is that it doesn't matter so much who's top or who's
43       or who's bottom, [uh:m although it- it may have=
44  P:                    [Sure.
45  C:   =some influence.
46  P:   Mm hm=
47  C:   =And that is that (.) the virus can travel both
48       wa:ys. [It's actually like in heterosexual sex=
49  P:          [Sure.
50  C:   =as we:ll.
51  P:   Mm [hm
52  C:      [But (.) m-men are (.) as (.) at much
53       risk (0.2) as women are:.
```

```
54  P:   Mm [hm
55  C:       [And the other way round.
56  P:   Okay:.=
57  C:   =Uh::m: (0.5) Although i- it's probably more
58       efficient in- in one directio:n [uh:m simply=
59  P:                                   [Yeah.
60  C:   =because (.) there is more of it obviously in
61       seme:n.
62  P:   Mm hm:
63  C:   Uh:m: (1.7) I- I think perhaps just to be clear now
64       our suggestion would be that if you're going to
65       continue to have a sexual relationship and there's
66       no reason why you shouldn't [.hhhh then=
67  P:                               [Mm hm
68  C:   =at this stage you: (0.2) should try to keep it as
69       safe as possible for a [variety of reasons. Some=
70  P:                          [Yeah.
71  C:   =people think that well .h assume we both have HIV
72       .h (0.2) it doesn't really matter then because we
73       can't infect one another with aids [with HIV=
74  P:                                       [Mm hm:
75  C:   =aga:in, well y'know that is so but there is a
76       problem with that thinking.=And that is .hhh if you
77       have unsafe sex (0.5) uh:m: (0.3) you- you ca:n get
78       a higher level of the virus in you,=you can be
79       reinoculated [with it. [(           )-
80  P:                [Okay:   [(Okay that)
81       (sounds-)][(Sure).
82  C:             [So that's one problem. .hhhh The other
83       is that (.) if either of you was carrying another
84       (.) sexually transmitted disease or perhaps
85       something else could be transmitted .hh hepatitis
86       (.) [gonorrhoea syphilis or something like that.=
87  P:       [Mm hm
88  C:   =.hhh It would trigger the immune system
89  P:   Mm hm:
90  C:   a:nd (.) if that happe:ns what happens is that the
91       virus replicates more rapidly.
92  P:   Mm hm:
93  C:   So: y-you get more virus. .hhhh So one way or the
94       other yeah you can have sex but (.) safer sex is
95       probably: uh[:m
96  P:               [Yeah:.. .h er[: What abou:t=
97  C:                             [(             )
98  P:   =er::: (0.6) oral sex without a condom. (0.2) er:
99       However::=
```

Extract 2 is taken from the pre-test counselling of a gay man whose partner has already tested positive. Notice how, unlike Extract 1, C begins the topic of sexual behaviour by asking a question of P rather than delivering advice. The question receives an answer (lines 3–7) which nicely reproduces the features of delay and generality that are recurrent in these interviews, irrespective of the sexual orientation of the patient (see Silverman and Bor, 1991).

Note now that, at line 13, C asks P to specify further that part of his answer that indicated a problem — 'not using a condom'. Only after P has gone into a detailed specification of what he and his partner are doing does C start to set up an advice package at line 41. In response, C receives only unmarked acknowledgments (e.g., 'sure' at line 44 and 'mm hm' at line 46). However, when C gives the reason for his advice, in terms of the dangers of unsafe sex even between two positive partners (lines 75–79), he gets an early, overlapping marked acknowledgment (Okay: [(Okay that)(sounds-)][(Sure) at line 80). Subsequent advice from C on lines 92–93 produces an overlapping question from P (lines 96–99). Together with a later question (not transcribed here) which refers to C's advice, this indicates considerable P uptake.

Although Extract 2 clearly supports Heritage and Sefi's point about how step-by-step advice sequences produce greater client uptake, it may be felt that, in comparing Extracts 1 and 2, we are not comparing like with like. More specifically, it could be argued that P's uptake of advice in 2 and lack of uptake in 1 may simply reflect that the patient in 2 was a gay man at high risk from a seropositive partner. This might have had two consequences. First, the greater uptake might not reflect how the advice package was set up but the possibility that this patient was paying more attention because he already had a perception of his own high risk of infection. Second, perhaps it is easier for counsellors to set up step-by-step advice sequences with gay men who come from a community already predisposed to take such advice seriously.

Nonetheless, our analysis suggests that the link between how advice is set up and client uptake holds whatever the gender or sexual orientation of the client. For instance, in an example where the client is a heterosexual young woman (Extract 4 below), we show how the step-by-step sequence is equally effective.

However, as we noted earlier, we should not overlook the deviant cases in our corpus of sequences. Extract 3 below is a counsellor-initiated advice sequence. Although P offers no newsworthiness tokens ('oh'), unexpectedly, there is plenty of P uptake, involving completion of C's turns (lines 3–4, 14 and 27) and references to the applicability of the advice to himself (20). Moreover, unlike Heritage and Sefi's findings, after lines 3–4, 14 and 27, the professional acknowledges her client's display of competence.

Extract 3

SW1–8A
```
 1   C:   But we can't tell you know whether uh one individual
 2        is going to or whether they're [no:t.
 3   P:                                    [(It's just on
 4        proportions).=
 5   C:   That's ri:[ght.
 6   P:             [(          )
 7   C:   .hhhh A:nd obviously if someone looks after
 8        themselves they stand a better chance you know
 9        keeping fit and healthy.
10   P:   Ye:s.
```

```
11  C:   .hhhh The advice we give is commonsense really if
12       you think about it.=To keep fit and healthy, (.)
13       eat a [well) a balanced di:et,
14  P:        [For your natural resistance.=
15  C:   =That's [right.
16  P:          [Ye:s.
17  C:   .hh Plenty of exerci:[se:
18  P:                       [Right.
19  C:   [Uh::m or enough exercise.
20  P:   [(I already get that) hheh .hhh [hhh .hhhh Too=
21  C:                                  [Yeah.
22  P:   =much of it. hhuh=
23  C:   =Enough slee:p.
24  P:   Y[es.
25  C:    [You know. All the things we should normally
26       do[: to keep healthy,
27  P:      [Right. Rather than let yourself get run down.=
28  C:   =That's ri:ght.
```

Extract 3 is remarkable for the large number of marked acknowledgments given by the client (lines 3–4, 14, 20, 22, and 27). How can we account for the far greater uptake in this than in Extract 1? After all, both involve truncated counsellor-initiated advice sequences.

Part of the answer seems to lie in the content of the advice given in each extract. Extract 3, unlike Extract 1, is largely concerned with what the counsellor tells people who have a positive test result. This leaves it open to the patient to treat what he is being told not as advice but as information-delivery (about the advice C would give if P turned out to be seropositive). However, if one looks back to Extract 1, the counsellor's depiction of the consequences of a negative test result might equally be heard as information-delivery rather than as specific advice to this patient. For instance, as in Extract 3, C avoids referring directly to P but uses the non-specific term 'someone'.

In both cases, then, we may be dealing with the uptake of what can be heard by the patient as information rather than advice. It follows that such uptake obviously need have no direct implication for what the patient does (as opposed to what he thinks), unlike the uptake of advice.

If Extracts 1 and 3 are similar in this respect, how can we account for the different kind of P uptake in each? The answer seems to be that in the Information-Delivery Format, unlike the Advice-Giving Format, patients are only interactionally required to give response tokens or unmarked acknowledgments (Perakyla and Silverman, 1991a). This means that in Information-Delivery it is *optional* whether patients offer marked acknowledgments. When they do so (as in Extract 3, via statements and displays of knowledge), they do not implicate themselves in any future lines of faction because they are only responding to what can be heard as information and not necessarily advice.

The optional character of the kind of patient uptake in Information-Delivery may account for the variance between Extracts 1 and 3. However, it does not explain why counsellors would want to package their advice in a way which makes patient uptake less likely. We shall argue that, by constructing advice sequences that can be heard as information-delivery, counsellors manage to stabilize advice-giving.

The Functions of Truncated Advice Sequences

In Extracts 1 and 3 we have seen examples of counsellors constructing what we might call 'hypothetical' advice sequences concerned with the advice the counsellor *would give* if '*someone*' (i.e., not necessarily this patient) had a particularly test result. A function of maintaining an ambiguous communication format is that the counsellor does not have to cope with the difficult interactional problems of the failure of patient uptake, given the instability of advice-giving. Through-out our corpus of examples counsellors exit quickly from personalized advice when patients offer only minimal response tokens or when they display overt resistance. A fascinating example of such resistance is found in two of our Trinidad extracts where patients overtly resist question-answer sequences about 'safer sex' by asserting that the counsellor should not be asking about their behaviour and know-ledge but, as the expert, telling them directly. Not only is advice-giving unstable but, if given in a step-by-step manner, it takes a long time (see Extract 4 below). Truncated, non-personalized advice sequences are usually far shorter — an important consideration for hard-pressed counsellors.

Another function of offering advice in this way is that it neatly handles many of the issues of delicacy that can arise in discussing sexual behaviour. First, the counsellor can be heard as making reference to what she tells 'anyone' so that this particular patient need not feel singled out for attention about his private life. Second, because there is no step-by-step method of questioning, patients are not required to expand on their sexual practices with the kinds of hesitations we shall see in Extract 4. Third, setting up advice sequences that can be heard as information-delivery shields the counsellor from some of the interactional difficulties of appearing to tell strangers what they should be doing in the most intimate aspects of their behaviour.

Practical Implications

Undoubtedly, there are gains for the counsellor in setting up advice packages which are truncated and non-personalized. Obviously, however, there are concomitant losses of proceeding this way. As we have shown, such advice packages produce far less patient uptake, and, therefore, their function in creating an environment in which people might re-examine their own sexual behaviour is distinctly problematic.

Two possible solutions suggest themselves from the data analyzed by this study. The first involves avoiding necessarily 'delicate' and unstable advice sequences but encouraging patients to draw their own conclusions from a particular line of questioning. A second approach, since both this method and step-by-step advice-giving take considerable time, involves finding ways of making more time available for more effective counselling.

Let us deal with the former idea first. Extract 4 below is an example of how a patient can construct her own 'advice' from a question-answer sequence. The extract occurs about thirty minutes into a consultation almost entirely based on C asking questions of P. This underlines the length of time that step-by-step methods can take. The extract begins with C requesting specification of P's problem-indicative response (giving up using condoms). Throughout, the symbol > indicates a passage that is important to our subsequent discussion.

Extract 4

4A.DG (38–9)

```
 1  C:   Well it's- so why did you decide then to stop using
 2       condoms er I mean er presumably you could have used
 3       both the pill and condoms. (.) Why did you actually
 4       decide to stop using condoms?
 5       (0.2)
 6  C:   D'you think.
 7       (0.7)
 8  P:   hhhh I don't really like using condoms. hheh I don't
 9       think anybody does. .hh (0.7) But I mean if I found
10       out (0.3) that I was HIV (.) negative (1.2) I: hhhh
11       I would with- with er: h my boyfriend now I would
12       start using them.=But If I: (0.2) broke up and
13       started seeing someone else I would (0.6) make sure
14       that I did. .hhh hhh=
15  C:>  =Ri:ght. (0.2) Do you think you're: (1.2) that you
16       feel happy then about (.) not using condoms with
17       him, (0.2) uhm d'you- d'you think that there
18       wouldn't be any risk. For example that he could not
19       be with any other partner (.) so you wouldn't have
20       to (0.5) (    [                    )
21  P:                 [I don't think he's sleeping
22       with anybody el[se.
23  C:                  [I was thinking I mean say you were
24       negative at the moment but he's positive.
25  P:   Mm
26       (0.5)
27  C:   And you decide to carry on and not using condoms,
28       (1.1)
29  P:   Yeah:?
30       (0.6)
31  C:   I'm wondering what you think i- d'you think it's
32       worthwhile taking that risk.
33       (0.8)
34  P:   .h[hh
35  C:     [Or: d'you [think it's not.=
36  P:                [We:ll
37  P:   =I've only go:t (.) I- I don't think I- I'm going to
38       start (.) I've got to finish this packet and then
39       I've got another packet to finish of the pill. (.)
40       Then after that I'm not taking any more:.
41       (0.9)
42  C:   .hh Right sorr[y but I meant about condoms.
43  P:                 [hhh
44       (.)
45  P:   Yeah. (.) So [(you know) when I'm not taking it=
46  C:                [I see.
47  P:   =a- when I'm not taking the pill any more: I will
48       use condoms.
```

```
49  C:>   .hh Right. I mean what if- what if (.) say you got
50          infected then in the next month while you'll still
51          taking the pi:lls (0.5) [and let's just say=
52  P:                              [Yeah (  )
53  C:    =he's positive (.) and you became infected (0.5)
54          what d'you think (.) if you could have (0.3) had
55          that experience agai:n how- how might things be
56          different do you think.
57  P:>   I would have u:sed .hh (0.2) used them.
58          (1.6)
59  (C):   .hhh
60          (0.8)
61  C:>   D'you know about anything else that you can use as
62          we:ll (0.2) as condoms to protect yourself or your
63          partners
64  P:    No I don't.
65  (C):   .hhh
66          (0.6)
67  C:    I mean condoms are a good thing because they
68          obviously are a barrier.=They actua[lly
69  P:                                          [Yeah:.
70          (0.2)
71  C:    form a barrier between you and the partner. And as
72          we said (0.2) HIV's in .hh in sem[en vaginal=
73  P:                                        [hhhh
74  C:    =secretions and (              ). .hhh But that's the
75          reason for using them whether it's vaginal
76          intercourse anal intercourse *may*be even oral se(h)x.
77  P:    Yeah:.=
78  C:    eh- eh- You know there's (.) potentially .hhhh (.)
79          uh- a possibility of .hhh transmission of body
80          flui:ds. .hhh *But* (.) we know condoms aren't a
81          hundred percent safe.=They slip off,=they rip. (0.3)
82          have you *a*ny idea what you could use as we:ll?
83          [That might help (.) back up the- .hh=
84  P:>   [A diaphragm?
85  C:    =certainly. .hh *That*'s a uh:m particularly the
86          cervix can be a fragile
87          (1.0)
88  P:    Ye[ah:.
89  C:      [orga:n that can: tear: .hh [and- and]=
90  P:                                  [So- so a]=
91  C:    =[(be an open side).
92  P:    =[diaphragm
93  P:>   is actually a- a way of protecting yourself (is)
94          (what you're [saying).
```

Just before this extract begins, the counsellor has elicited a statement from the patient that she has stopped using condoms with her present boyfriend. Given this problem-indicative response, C follows it up in the usual step-by-step manner, by asking P to specify her answer (lines 1–6). P's specification is addressed to the future circumstances in which she would use condoms even though she does not like them (lines 8–14). At this point, instead of offering advice, C uses a leading question (lines 15–20, marked >) which asks P to think about the risks of her present behaviour. When P's answers to this and further questions still do not elicit from P a commitment to change her behaviour at once, C changes tack. At lines 49–57 (>), C invites P to imagine a possible future in which she had been infected because her boyfriend had been HIV-positive. P now says she would use condoms. Having elicited that hypothetical commitment from P, C asks about what other forms of protection she might use (lines 61–63 >). When P say she doesn't know, C continues the topic until P herself produces the item (84>). Beautifully, then (at 90–94 >), P produces the advice as a summary of the argument present in C's questions and statements.

Note two nice features of this sequence. First, an advice summary by a patient is one of the strongest marked acknowledgments of a professional's advice that one sees. Second, this summary is produced in a local context where the counsellor has not actual delivered and direct advice, other than underlining some of what his patient has said.

Extract 4 thus shows how considerable uptake may be achieved by a full sequence without any explicit advice. However, in common with many consultations at this clinic, this interview lasts about forty-five minutes. Staff at other centres might argue that this is an impracticable way to use their time and resources.

There is, therefore, a need to explore other means to give more time to counsellors. One possibility that British centres might consider following is the US model of group pre-test counselling combined with the completion by patients of individual, confidential questionnaires about their reasons for wanting an HIV test. This is then followed by lengthy one-to-one counselling at the *post-test* stage. A second possibility is to retain pre-test individual counselling but to make more use of the time while patients are waiting. Interactive videos, although costly in the short run, might well turn out be cost-efficient in terms of covering a lot of the ground currently taken up by information-delivery by the counsellor. Not only would this allow each counselling session to be more structured to the needs to individual patients but it would also make pre-test counselling far less repetitive and far less boring for the counsellor.

Conclusions

Despite Nelkin's (1987, p. 982) call for studies 'to evaluate diverse means of communicating information about sex', one is struck by the lack of research on the actual process of HIV counselling. As Bor (1989, p. 184) has noted, research so far has concentrated on 'approaches to behavioural change, health education and psychosocial support rather than communication in clinical settings.'

Faced with this lack of knowledge, our study supports Green's (1989) assertion that most counsellors have adopted a largely pragmatic approach. Counselling practice varies from one centre to another. Moreover, our research shows that there is no one-to-one coincidence between any one way of setting up advice and any individual counsellor. Certainly, particular counsellors do tend to use one advice format as their home base and, overwhelmingly, this involves a truncated sequence of counsellor-initiated advice. Yet even the most directive counsellors do occasionally try step-by-step advice sequences.

The research has shown the practical skills of counsellors. For instance, by using truncated sequences, they at least manage to produce relatively short counselling sessions with minimal overt conflict. Given the time pressures many of them face, this is no mean achievement. With greater knowledge of what is effective in HIV counselling, and better organization of time and other resources, there is thus some prospect of future modifications to counselling practice in this area. Following Miller and Bor's (1988) text on HIV/AIDS counselling, our research has revealed the nature and effectiveness of step-by-step methods of counselling based on question-answer sequences rather than on the delivery of information. Through such methods clients do indeed learn *relevant* information. More important, following Stoller and Rutherford (1989), they learn the skills to determine what is appropriate for themselves and their partners.

Acknowledgements

An earlier version of this paper was given at a staff seminar, Department of Sociology, University of California, Los Angeles on 5 February 1991. We should like to thank John Heritage and Anssi Perakyla for their invaluable comments and suggestions. We are also most grateful to the counsellors and patients whose conversations are reported here and to the Health Education Authority and Glaxo Holdings plc for funding this research.

Note

1   For an example of how we have transcribed and analyzed video-tapes of counselling, see Perakyla and Silverman (1991b).

References

AGGLETON, P. (1989) 'Evaluating Health Education about AIDS', in P. AGGLETON, P. DAVIES and G. HART (Eds), *AIDS: Social Representations, Social Practices*, Lewes, Falmer Press.

BECK, E., *et al.* (1987) 'HIV Testing: Changing Trends at a Clinic for Sexually Transmitted Diseases', *British Medical Journal*, 295, pp. 191–3.

BOR, R. (1989) 'AIDS Counselling', *AIDS CARE*, 1, 2, pp. 184–7.

CARBALLO, M. and MILLER, D. (1989) 'HIV Counselling: Problems and Opportunities in Defining the New Agenda for the 1990's', *AIDS Care*, 1, 2, pp. 117–23.

FENTON, T. (1987) 'AIDS and Psychiatry: practical, social and ethical issues', *Journal of the Royal Society of Medicine*, 80, pp. 271–5.

FITZPATRICK, R., *et al.* (1986) 'Survey of Psychological Disturbance in Patients Attending a Sexually Transmitted Diseases Clinic', *Genitourinary Medicine*, 62, pp. 111–15.

GOEDERT, J. (1987) 'What Is Safe Sex? Suggested Standards Linked to Testing for Human Immunodeficiency Virus', *New England Journal of Medicine*, 316, 21, pp. 1339–42.

GREEN, J. (1989) 'Counselling for HIV Infection and AIDS: The Past and the Future', *AIDS Care*, 1, 1, pp. 5–10.

GREENBLAT, C., *et al.* (1989) 'An Innovative Programme of Counselling Family Members and Friends of Seropositive Haemophiliacs', *AIDS Care*, 1, 1, pp. 67–75.

HENRY, K. (1988) 'Setting AIDS Priorities: The Need for a Closer Alliance of Public

Health and Clinical Approaches towards the Control of AIDS', *American Journal of Public Health*, 78, 9, pp. 1210–12.

HERITAGE, J. and SEFI, S. (forthcoming) 'Dilemmas of Advice: Aspects of the Delivery and Reception of Advice in Interactions between Health Visitors and First Time Mothers', in P. DREW and J. HERITAGE (Eds), *Talk at Work*, Cambridge, Cambridge University Press.

HODGKIN, P. (1988) 'HIV Infection: The Challenge to General Practitioners', *British Medical Journal*, 296, pp. 516–17.

MILLER, D. (1987) 'Counselling', *British Medical Journal*, 294, pp. 1671–4.

MILLER, D. (1988) 'HIV and Social Psychiatry', *British Medical Bulletin*, 44, 1, pp. 130–48.

MILLER, D. and BOR, R. (1988) AIDS: *A Guide to Clinical Counselling*, London, Science Press.

MILLER, D. and PINCHING, A.J. (1989) 'HIV Tests and Counselling: Current Issues', *AIDS*, 3, Supplement 1, S187–93.

MILLER, D., *et al.* (1986) 'Organising a Counselling Service for Problem Related to AIDS', *Genitourinary Medicine*, 62, pp. 116–22.

MITCHELL, J.C. (1983) 'The Logic of the Analysis of Social Situations and Cases', *Sociological Review*, 31, 2, pp. 187–211.

NELKIN, D. (1987) 'AIDS and the Social Sciences: Review of Useful Knowledge and Research Needs', *Reviews of Infectious Diseases*, 9, 5, pp. 980–7.

PERAKYLA, A. and BOR, R. (1990) 'Interactional Problems of Addressing "Dreaded Issues" in HIV-Counselling', *AIDS Care*, 2, 4, pp. 325–38.

PERAKYLA, A. and SILVERMAN, D. (1991a) 'Reinterpreting Speech-Exchange Systems: Communication Formats in AIDS Counselling', *Sociology*, 25, 4, pp. 627–651.

PERAKYLA, A. and SILVERMAN, D. (1991b) 'Owning the Experience of Others', *Text*, 11, 3, pp. 441–80.

PETERMAN, T. and CURRAN, J. (1986) 'Sexual Transmission of Human Immunodeficiency Virus', *Journal of the American Medical Association*, 256, 16, pp. 2222–6.

QUINN, T. (1988) 'Human Immunodeficiency Virus Infection among Patients Attending Clinics for Sexually Transmitted Diseases', *The New England Journal of Medicine*, 318, 4, pp. 197–203.

RICHARDS, T. (1986) 'Don't Tell Me on a Friday', *British Medical Journal*, 292, p. 943.

SACKS, H. (1974) 'On the Analyzability of Stories by Children', in R. TURNER (Ed.), *Ethnomethodology*, Harmondsworth, Penguin Books.

SACKS, H., *et al.* (1974) 'A Simplest Systematics for the Analysis of Turn-Taking in Conversation', *Language*, 50, pp. 696–735.

SADLER, C. (1988) 'Sexually Transmitted Diseases: More than Tea and Sympathy', *Nursing Times*, 84, 49, pp. 30–2.

SALT, H., *et al.* (1989) 'Paradoxical Interventions in Counselling for People with an Intractable AIDS-Worry', *AIDS Care*, 1, 1, pp. 39–44.

SHERNOFF, M. (1988) 'Integrating Safer-Sex Counselling into Social Work Practice', *Social Casework*, June, pp. 334–9.

SHERR, L. (1989) 'Health Education', *AIDS Care*, 1, 2, pp. 188–92.

SILVERMAN, D. (1985) *Qualitative Methodology and Sociology*, Aldershot, Gower.

SILVERMAN, D. (1990) 'The Social Organization of Counselling', in P. AGGLETON, P. DAVIES and G. HART, (Eds) *AIDS: Individual, Cultural and Policy Dimensions*, Lewes Falmer Press.

SILVERMAN, D. and BOR, R. (1991) 'The Delicacy of Describing Sexual Partners in HIV-Test Counselling: Implications for Practice', *Counselling Psychology Quarterly*, 4, 2/3, pp. 177–190.

SILVERMAN, D. and PERAKYLA, A. (1990) 'AIDS Counselling: The Interactional Organization of Talk about "Delicate" Issues', *Sociology of Health and Illness*, 12, 3, pp. 293–318.

SONNEX, C., *et al.* (1987) 'HIV Infection: Increase in Public Awareness and Anxiety', *British Medical Journal*, 295, pp. 193–5.

STOLLER, E.J. and RUTHERFORD, G.W. (1989) 'Evaluation of AIDS Prevention and Control Programs', *AIDS*, 3, Supplement 1, S289–96.

THOMPSON, C. and MCIVER, A. (1988) 'HIV Counselling: Change in Trends in Public Concern', *Health Bulletin*, 46, pp. 237–45.

WATNEY, S. (1987) *Policing Desire*, London, Methuen.

WORLD HEALTH ORGANIZATION (1988) *Guidelines for the Development of a National AIDS Prevention and Control Programme*, WHO AIDS Series 1, Geneva.

Appendix: The Transcription Symbols

*	* What?	Invented example.
[	C2: quite a [while Mo: [yea	Left brackets indicate the point at which a current speaker's talk is overlapped by another's talk.

=	W: that I'm aware of
	    =
	C: =Yes. Would you
	    confirm that?
		Equal signs, one at the end of the line and one at the beginning, indicate no gap between the two lines.

(.4)	Yes (.2) yeah	Numbers in parentheses indicate elapsed time in silence in tenths of a second.
(.)	to get (.) treatment	A dot in parentheses indicates a tiny gap, probably no more than one-tenth of a second.
	What's *up?*	Italic type indicates some form of stress, via pitch and/or amplitude.
::	O:*kay?*	Colons indicate prolongation of the immediately prior sound. The length of the row of colons indicates the length of the prolongation.
WORD	I've got ENOUGH TO WORRY ABOUT	Capitals, except at the beginnings of lines, indicate especially loud sounds relative to the surrounding talk.
.hhhh	I feel that (.2) .hhh	A row of h's prefixed by a dot indicates an inbreath; without a dot, an outbreath. The length of the row of h's indicates the length of the in- or outbreath.
( )	future risks and ( ) and life ( )	Empty parentheses indicate the transcriber's inability to hear what was said.
(word)	Would you see (there) anything positive	Parenthesized words are possible hearings.
(( ))	confirm that ((continues))	Double parentheses contain author's descriptions rather than transcriptions.

14 The Voluntary Sector, Gay Men and HIV/AIDS

Kathy McCann

Voluntary groups have long provided basic services in Britain, and it is not surprising that many such organizations were either established or changed their focus in response to HIV infection and AIDS (Green, 1989). An active voluntary sector is supported by central government both generally in the context of providing care in the community and more specifically in relation to HIV and AIDS. The recent White Paper, 'Caring for People: Community Care in the Next Decade', for example, stated that service plans should include making 'the maximum possible use of private and voluntary providers, so as to increase the available range of options and widen consumer choice' (HMSO, 1989, 1.11). In relation to HIV and AIDS, and in 1986, after visiting America, the then Secretary of State for Health, Norman Fowler, praised the model of care available in San Francisco, arguing that it was suitable for Britain to adopt. This model relies on non-profit-making groups providing the majority of services.

Voluntary organizations in Britain have already been responsible for campaigning for those affected by HIV, coordinating approaches around specific issues, self-help, and actively providing services, often in integrated and innovative ways (Schramm-Evans, 1990; Weeks, 1990; Green, 1989).

Using data from semi-structured interviews with 265 gay men who were HIV antibody positive, this chapter reports on respondents' use of a number of voluntary agencies and describes their views on how they operate. The focus is on the services used by a group of gay men, mostly in London. It does not provide either an exhaustive list of help available from non-statutory organizations or a list of the many agencies which exist in relation to HIV or AIDS. Nevertheless, the account which these men gave of their use of voluntary organizations offers valuable insight into the actual and potential role of such agencies in supporting people who are HIV antibody positive, the association between being a volunteer and receiving help, and the relationship of different organizations to each other and to statutory services.

Background and Methods

Questions about voluntary organizations were included as part of a wider study in which HIV antibody positive gay men attending a London teaching hospital

Table 1   How Would You Contact a Voluntary Group If You Needed To? (percentages)

Already have telephone number	39
Get telephone number from British Telecom/or write	13
Drop in	2
From gay press	23
From friends	8
Through doctor in clinic	4
Through clinic notices	10
Ask community liaison team	6
Ask other professionals	5
Other	3

Notes: N = 171, i.e., the number of people at second interview. More than one response was possible.

were asked about the use, views and experiences of a variety of health, social and lay services. Respondents were recruited through the hospital's genito-urinary and immunology outpatient clinics and through the designated ward for the care of people with HIV/AIDS between November 1988 and June 1989. Personal interviews took place with 265 individuals, 86 per cent of those who expressed interest in the study, by completing a form included in a letter about the study. Second interviews were carried out with 65 per cent of the original group six to ten months later. Three per cent of respondents were lost to further interview because they had moved (mostly abroad), 16 per cent because they had died and 11 per cent because they could not subsequently be contacted. Five per cent refused to participate in a follow-up interview.

The whole spectrum of HIV disease was represented, from being unsymptomatic to having a diagnosis of AIDS. Because four people were too ill to complete the full interview, the responses of only 261 people are reported here. Changes over time are based on the 171 second interviews. Of the original group interviewed, 66 per cent were working, the majority full-time. Just under half (47 per cent) were professionals or had intermediate occupations (social classes I or II). Forty-five per cent owned their own accommodation, and 40 per cent lived alone.

Ease of Access to Voluntary Organizations

One important aspect of any agency or service is the ease with which people can make contact with it. During the second interview we asked how easy or difficult people would find it to contact a voluntary organization if they needed help; only 5 per cent felt they would have problems. Table 1 summarizes the ways in which people said they anticipated making contact with a voluntary agency. Other responses included getting in touch via an intermediary, through the citizens' advice bureau, through a local authority or through advertisements. Just under a quarter (24 per cent) said they would use a professional or statutory service to facilitate contact.

Use of Voluntary Organizations

One of the early functions of voluntary organizations working in the field of HIV/AIDS was to provide both oral and written information (Schramm-Evans, 1990). When asked where they had obtained their initial information about HIV, 17 per cent of people in the study reported reading a leaflet; many of the leaflets were produced by or with the help of voluntary groups. A further 8 per cent said they received information directly from the Terrence Higgins Trust (THT) and 2 per cent from other voluntary groups including Body Positive (BP) and the London Lighthouse (LL).

At a later date, and after they knew they were HIV antibody positive, 177 of the men (68 per cent) had had some additional contact by the time of their first interview, and a further twenty-one by their second. Three-quarters of respondents overall had had some contact with voluntary organizations at some time.

Because voluntary organizations rely to some degree on individuals providing their labour free, it was not surprising that people combined being a volunteer with receiving help from an agency. A small proportion of respondents worked exclusively as a volunteer without receiving help (8 per cent); just over half (56 per cent) received help only; and the remainder both worked for an organization and received help (24 per cent). Twelve per cent had a single or infrequent contact.

Those who received help were more likely to have experienced poor health (84 per cent compared to 57 per cent of those who did not receive help), though there were no other differences in any other personal characteristics of those in touch with the voluntary organizations and those not. This included whether or not respondents had withheld information about the HIV status from others, or whether they lived alone.

As would be expected from a relatively inclusive sample, the kinds of assistance people obtained from voluntary organizations varied enormously. Some people simply maintained contact through newsletters, occasional meetings or socials, others received information and advice, while others gained counselling support and/or practical physical help. The following comments reflect the different degrees of involvement:

> I was introduced to BP people while I was in hospital. It was literally to say help was available.

> I once phoned them to recommend a dentist and they did.

> I had help with moving and social security advice from Frontliners.

> I received financial help in a general way from Crusaid.

> They helped with a small grant to help me buy a fridge and double bed.

> A buddy (from THT) helps with shopping, keeps me company, he's good entertainment and a nice friend.

At the first interview twenty-four people said they were receiving regular support from a volunteer at home, and an additional thirteen were being visited

Table 2   Presence of Informal Carer and Contact with Voluntary Organizations

| | Informal care contact (percentages) | | |
	Yes	No	All
THT	57	43*	48
BP	41	38	39
FL	35	18**	25
LL	19	19	19
IM	13	2**	6
Financial	6	4	5
Telephone	5	6	5
Other	12	10	10
N (=100%)	104	157	261

Notes: *p < 0.05.
          **p < 0.001.

by the second interview. Half were seeing their 'buddy' at least once a week, and almost all felt that the assistance they received was very or fairly helpful. Slightly more of those that had a buddy — thirty-nine (15 per cent) — felt they would have liked the support of a volunteer at home but were without it. However, only one in five (21 per cent) of these people had asked for such help.

The Organizations

In the course of the study we obtained information about different voluntary organizations and two self-help organizations offering information and support. Forty-eight per cent of people were in touch with THT and 39 per cent with BP. A quarter of respondents had had contact with Frontliners (FL), a self-help group especially for people with AIDS; 19 per cent had had contact with LL, an organization offering respite and terminal care, counselling and general support; and 6 per cent had had contact with Immunity (IM), a group offering legal advice. Finally, agencies offering financial help or help over the telephone were each mentioned by 5 per cent of the group. Ten per cent named other organizations, including specific local agencies and those for drug users. There were no age or class differences in whether people were in touch with the different voluntary organizations or not. Those in touch with THT, BP or IM may, however, have been more likely to live alone, although these differences were not statistically significant. Those who had an informal carer were also more likely to be involved with the voluntary organizations in general and THT, BP and IM in particular (see Table 2).

As would be expected, there was a relationship between people's health and the organizations they had contacted. This was clearly related to the organization's function. Thus those in contact with FL were significantly more likely to have a diagnosis of AIDS or ARC than were those in touch with THT or BP (75 per cent compared to 49 and 41 per cent respectively). People who had contacted Immunity were more likely to have experienced poor health than those who had not (44 per cent compared to 15 per cent of those not in touch). (See Table 3.)

Table 3   Voluntary Organization Contact by Diagnostic Status

| | Diagnosis of ARC/AIDS (percentages) | | |
	Yes	No	All
THT	65	39*	48
BP	45	38	39
FL	51	10*	25
LL	23	17	19
IM	13	3*	6
Financial	11	2*	5
Telephone	4	6	5
Other	13	9	10
N (=100%)	95	166	261

Note: *p < 0.001.

Table 4   Relationship between Contact with One Organization and Another

| | Proportion of people who are also in contact with each of the other organizations (percentages) | | | | |
	THT	BP	FL	LL	All
THT	—	71	89	68	48
BP	57	—	69	68	39
FL	45	43	—	44	19
LL	27	33	34	—	25
N (=100%)	126	102	64	50	261

Note: Organizations used by fewer than fifty people are not included as the numbers in each cell become too small.

In many circumstances people used more than one organization. Two-thirds of those who had used one voluntary organization had used at least one other; one in five had had contact with three; and 8 per cent had links with five different ones. Table 4 indicates the relationship between use of different agencies.

Although some of the organizations have apparently similar aims, respondents often had contact with more than one, which on the surface was indicative of some duplication in the use of agencies. However, from the comments which were made, it was apparent that different organizations were used in a complementary way to meet a variety of needs:

> THT gave me lots of advice when I had a legal problem at work, FL gave advice on individual benefits. BP, I used to be involved in hospital visits and telephone counselling. Telephone advice from THT and FL, newsletter from Body Positive. Christmas card and social worker from LL.

This complementarity also characterized circumstances where a respondent worked as a volunteer and received help.

THT gave me a one-off grant, BP gave me counselling when I was first diagnosed as HIV positive. They were the first people I turned to when I was first diagnosed. I've done some fundraising from them.

FL, I registered with them so I could find out what facilities were available from the Department of Social Security and the local authority and they put me in touch with a coordinator. I have raised money for LL.

There were no significant changes in the combinations of agencies used between the first and second interviews, although there were increases in use of some over the ten-month period. This was particularly true for FL, LL and Immunity. These increases reflect changes in the health of those newly using these agencies, and in the case of the LL, at least, is a probable reflection of an expansion in the services it offered over this time. Three people had received financial support for the first time, and eleven people had received help over the telephone. Forty-six people had become involved in the work of voluntary organizations by the time we interviewed them again, although previously they had mostly only had a single contact.

Involvement in the Work of Voluntary Organizations

In San Francisco, where much community care is provided by volunteers, one of the great concerns had been whether there would be sufficient people with enough energy to sustain the many initiatives already established (McCann, 1990). This concern must also be relevant to non-paid volunteer care in Britain. Indeed, one man in the study illustrated a reason likely to cause 'burn-out' when he explained why he was no longer involved:

I became very aware of what might happen to me if I became ill and also meeting other people who are HIV positive. I am no longer involved as I can no longer cope with the loss of people I've become so fond of.

Why people are motivated to become involved, how they do so, and what they get out of it, are useful to an understanding of how people's volunteer activity is maintained. Reasons why people began working as volunteers included the view that it was a means of repaying the help given to themselves or others. As two respondents put it:

It was to provide a useful memorial when my lover died.

I feel I'm giving them back to say thank you for what they did when I needed them.

Alternatively, altruism was an often cited response: 'One feels a sort of civic duty — I obviously can't give blood in the normal way as I used to — so I help in a small way.' For others, volunteering reduced their isolation and provided positive social contact:

It keeps my feet on the ground, made me feel I wasn't alone with the virus and I have made a lot of contacts with people in the same situation.

It breaks down the isolation. I like to think I'm helping someone and they're helping me. I'm meeting good interesting people.

Initially they were a source of information, then came fund raising. I've manned the telephones for them on occasion, had a lot of moral support and it's a social outlet as well, meeting others who are body positive.

For others, involvement with a voluntary agency kept them active and was pleasurable:

It occupies my mind and I'm helping other people. I feel better for that.

It makes me feel valued and gives me a lot of pleasure.

For yet others it was linked to self-help:

It gives me something to do for a couple of days a week and a lot to complain about.

[I became involved through] asking and not finding. They did not have the information I wanted. I then found it and this got me involved.

It's part of feeling that something has to be done, you just can't sit back and not get involved.

Giving and receiving help at the same time filling gaps in my life. They need HIV positive people to react and can understand fears. I get more out of the work than I give to it.

Basically with the general attitude of the public about AIDS it's good to see a group of people get together and realize that they won't be ignored.

Voluntary Sector Involvement and Its Relation to Statutory Care

There were some connections between respondents' involvement with the voluntary organizations and their contact with services in the public sector, yet many of these relationships disappeared or changed when the person's experience of illness was taken into account. Following a log linear analysis of the relationship between contact with volunteers and the use of services, taking into account the possibility that the relationship itself might be confounded by illness, only an increased likelihood of seeing a psychologist ($X^2 = 9.203$ (1df) $p < .01$) and a dietitian ($X^2 = 3.85$ (1df) $p < .05$) was found to be associated with contact with voluntary organizations. A relationship, but in the opposite direction, appeared between home help and contact with volunteers for those with a diagnosis of AIDS or ARC such that where a volunteer was involved, the home help was less likely to be. All other relationships disappeared when illness was controlled for, suggesting that people were no more or less likely to use statutory services if they were also in touch with volunteers but instead that, where they are used, this is probably in conjunction with each other.

A similar log linear model was used to assess the relationship between use of statutory services and volunteers, taking into account whether the respondent had nominated an informal carer. Here no relationships were found to exist. However, fewer people who had an informal carer and a diagnosis of AIDS or ARC were in touch with a voluntary organization, although the difference here was not significant (56 compared to 60 per cent).

Reasons for Not Asking for Help

A quarter of respondents had not had any contact with any of the agencies. The main reasons for this were apparent from the responses. First, people felt that contact was inappropriate for them personally, although most did not rule out the possibility of obtaining help in the future should they require it, as the following comments indicate:

> I've never yet felt the need of support. If I got seriously ill I would go to them, if I wanted to talk to someone face to face.

> I feel guilty about not using them but I really don't need help.

> Pleased they are there for others. I would have no hesitation in using them if I needed to.

> I'm fit and don't need it. If I were ill I'd be grateful.

The other reasons given for not using voluntary groups included the groups they were perceived as catering for:

> I'm not an open gay man — you need to be to go to these places.

> I've never been on the gay scene. I have nothing in common with them.

Also, it was felt that contact with them might involve inadvertent disclosure of their HIV status to others — 'I'd have to be desperate to ask for local help' — or it was anticipated that to make contact would somehow be depressing: 'I think it would make me very depressed if you go and people are ill'; or simply because: 'I haven't yet got the courage.'

Discussion

Volunteers played a considerable part in supporting people with HIV infection in the present study. Three-quarters of the group had been in touch with a voluntary agency at some time. Only a small proportion (5 per cent) anticipated any difficulty in contacting them if the need should arise. A quarter of these said they would use professionals to achieve contact, suggesting the importance of maintaining links between the two.

Although 14 per cent of respondents had a volunteer visiting them at home, more (15 per cent) said they would have liked to have had this option, even though only one in five had asked. There may be some scope here to ensure that access to existing services is more readily available, and where such a service does not exist, for increased funding to be allocated to this kind of work. In general terms the only characteristic which made it more likely for people to be in touch with volunteers was that they had experienced ill health. In the use of individual agencies the clearest pattern emerged in relation to contact with IM, which was used more often once people became ill. This suggests that legal advice may be more often required by people at a later stage, to get their affairs in order or to sort out difficulties resulting from ill health. Use of switchboards and telephone helplines was more likely for those without any HIV-related symptoms, which is perhaps unremarkable as it is often at an early stage that the kind of information and support given by a switchboard may be perceived to be most useful.

Two-thirds of people were in touch with more than one organization. While the relationship between illness and contact with the different groups (which was largely explained by the function of the organization) might explain some of the overlap, differences still remained, and though it is conceivable that some duplication exists, the respondents' accounts suggest that, on an individual basis at least, different agencies were being used in a complementary way. The fact that people were using different organizations with similar functions perhaps indicates a need to review whether organizations could cooperate more extensively to rationalize their functions, or whether the range of choice would be adversely affected if this were to happen.

Respondents often combined working for an organization with receiving help from the voluntary sector. Reasons for involvement in volunteer work varied but included self-help, altruism, giving them something to do and that it was sociable. The contributions which these volunteers made to the organizations were sizeable and represent a community response, arising because existing systems did not work (Weeks, 1990). Moreover, this involves the *gay* community because it is within this community that HIV first appeared, and it was from within this community that the first self-help responses emerged. It must be asked, however, how far this level of commitment can be maintained. There was some evidence that because some of the organizations were identified with the gay community, they were not used as widely as might have been anticipated. This reluctance on the part of some gay men raises questions about how far these organizations should be expected to adapt to provide services to all those with HIV infection on their own terms, and, if so, how this could occur.

Few independent associations between contact with agencies and use of statutory services existed. Only use of a psychologist and the dietitian was linked to respondents' involvement with volunteers. This suggests that rather than volunteers substituting for statutory services or statutory services for volunteers, the two are used in conjunction. The only exception existed in relation to the use of home helps. Here an inverse relationship existed: volunteers were more likely to be visiting the person at home when a home help was not.

It appears from this study that voluntary organizations have provided choice and an addition to statutory services. It has also been argued that they can react more quickly than statutory services which may find it harder to adapt to changing needs. Moreover, voluntary groups may be more empathetic and, because of their origins in self-help, may be more able to provide appropriate and acceptable care (Green, 1990; McCann, 1990).

Recent UK government statements have stressed the importance of voluntary organizations in providing community care in general, thus affording consumers greater choice. The experience of respondents in the present study indicates that such organizations fulfilled a role for them, separate from the public sector, providing access to and choice of a greater variety of services. There is a danger in areas such as HIV, where the role of voluntary organizations is clearly successful, that too heavy reliance will be placed upon them in the future to provide flexible, empathetic and innovative services rather than for statutory services to be encouraged to be more responsive, and user-friendly themselves. Voluntary organizations undoubtedly lessen the economic impact of health and social care by providing both alternative and fundamental care; as such, they can be taken advantage of as 'care on the cheap'. There are intrinsic limits to this dependency on unpaid labour (Arno, 1989; McCann, 1990). Efforts need to be made to get the balance and co-existence of the two systems correct, as well as the funding position. This is important both in terms of what it is possible or appropriate for each to provide and in terms of what is desirable from the point of view of the range of care available for clients and their satisfaction.

References

ARNO, P.S. (1989) 'The Non-Profit Making Sectors' Response to the AIDS Epidemic: Community-based Services in San Francisco', *American Journal of Public Health*, 76, pp. 1325–30.

GREEN, J. (1989) 'The Role of Voluntary Groups in the Community', in J. GREEN and A. McCREANER (Eds), *Counselling in HIV Infection and AIDS*, Oxford, Blackwell Scientific Publications.

HMSO (1989) *Caring for People: Community Care in the Next Decade and Beyond*, London, HMSO, Cmnd 849.

McCANN, K. (1990) 'Care in the Community by the Community', *AIDS Care*, 2, 4, pp. 421–4.

SCHRAMM-EVANS, Z. (1990) 'Responses to AIDS 1986–1987', in P. AGGLETON, P. DAVIS and G. HART (Eds), *AIDS: Individual, Cultural and Policy Dimensions*, Lewes, Falmer Press.

WEEKS, J. (1988) 'Love in a Cold Climate', in P. AGGLETON and H. HOMANS (Eds), *Social Aspects of AIDS*, Lewes, Falmer Press.

WEEKS, J. (1990) 'Post Modern AIDS?', in T. BOFFIN and S. GUPTA (Eds), *Estatic Antibodies: Resisting the AIDS Mythology*, London, Rivers Oram Press.

Notes on Contributors

Peter Aggleton is Director of the Health and Education Research Unit at Goldsmiths' College, University of London. He is a director of a number of major projects concerned with HIV/AIDS health promotion. His recent publications include *Nursing Models and the Nursing Process* (with Helen Chalmers, Macmillan, 1986), *Deviance* (Tavistock, 1987), *Social Aspects of AIDS* (ed. with Hilary Homans, Falmer, 1988), *AIDS: Social Representations and Social Practices* (ed. with Graham Hart and Peter Davies, Falmer, 1989), *Health* (Routledge, 1990), *AIDS: Individual, Cultural and Policy Dimensions* (ed. with Graham Hart and Peter Davies, Falmer, 1990) and *AIDS: Responses, Interventions and Care* (ed. with Graham Hart and Peter Davies, Falmer, 1991).

Don Baxter is the Executive Director of the AIDS Council of New South Wales, the largest non-government AIDS organization in Australia. The Council conducts a wide range of HIV/AIDS education, care, support and advocacy programmes. He was instrumental in establishing the Social Aspects of the Prevention of AIDS project, the joint research programme between Macquarie University and the AIDS Council. He is a member of the New South Wales Ministerial Advisory Committee on AIDS, and for four years served on the Australian National Council on AIDS.

Rigmor Berg is a recipient of a Commonwealth AIDS Research Grant Post-Graduate Award and is currently working part-time as a research and evaluation consultant.

Virginia Berridge is Senior Lecturer and Co-Director of the AIDS Social History Programme at the London School of Hygiene and Tropical Medicine. Her publications include *Opium and the People: Opiate Use in Nineteenth Century England* (Yale, 1987); Health and Disease in *The Cambridge Social History of Britain; Drugs Research and Policy in Britain: A Review of the 1980s* (Gower, 1990) and articles on the history of AIDS policies in the UK.

Robert Bor is Senior Lecturer in Psychology at City University, London. Between 1987 and 1991 he was Principal Clinical Psychologist and District AIDS Counsellor, Royal Free Hospital, London. He is the author (with Riva Miller) of *AIDS: A Guide to Clinical Counselling* (Science Press, 1988) and around fifty papers in academic and professional journals on aspects of AIDS counselling.

Bob Connell is 1991–92 Professor of Australian Studies at Harvard University. Since 1976 he has been foundation Professor of Sociology at Macquarie University in Sydney. His books include *Class Structure in Australian History* (with T.H. Irving, Longman Cheshire, 1980), *Making the Difference* (with D.J. Ashenden, S. Kessler and G.W. Dowsett, Allen and Unwin, 1982), *Which Way is Up?* (Allen and Unwin, 1983) *Teachers' Work* (Allen and Unwin, 1985), *Gender and Power: Society, Families and Social Division* (Allen and Unwin; Polity Press) and *Staking a Claim: Feminism, Bureaucracy and the State*, (with S. Franzway and D. Court, Allen and Unwin; Polity Press, 1989). *Running Twice as Hard*, a study of the Disadvantaged Schools Program in Australia, is in press.

June Crawford is Senior Lecturer in the School of Behavioural Sciences, Macquarie University. She has long experience in designing and analyzing surveys, many in health-related areas. For the past four years she has been involved in AIDS prevention research, in theorizing feminist psychology and in research on women's health and community participation in health.

Peter Davies is Lecturer in Sociology at Essex University. He is a Principal Investigator of Project SIGMA (Socio-sexual Investigations of Gay Men and AIDS) and author of *Key Texts in Multidimensional Scaling* (Heinemann, 1982), *Images of Social Stratification* (Sage, 1985). He is editor (with Peter Aggleton and Graham Hart) of *AIDS: Social Representations, Social Practices* (Falmer, 1989), *AIDS: Individual, Cultural and Policy Dimensions* (Falmer, 1990) and *AIDS: Responses, Interventions and Care* (Falmer, 1991).

Mark Davis is Research Assistant in the AIDS Research Unit, School of Behavioural Sciences, Macquarie University. He has mostly worked on the Class, Homosexuality and AIDS Prevention and Functional Injecting Drug Users Projects co-ordinating fieldwork, conducting qualitative interviews and analysis. He previously worked for the Australian Federation of AIDS Organisations as a peer educator with gay and bisexual men.

Gary Dowsett is Research Fellow in Sociology at Macquarie University. For the last five years he has worked full-time in HIV/AIDS research, coordinating a series of social research projects on the responses of gay men and other homosexually active men to HIV/AIDS. His current research interests are focused on an investigation of the relationship of homosexuality, gender and class. He is also Vice-President of the AIDS Council of New South Wales, Australia.

François Fleury has coordinated various HIV/AIDS prevention studies among migrant groups in Switzerland, particularly among Turkish asylum seekers. A psychotherapist, he has considerable transcultural research experience, and has given numerous presentations in the fields of ethnopsychiatry, migration and mental health.

Richard Freeman is Lecturer in Social Policy in the Department of Political Science and Social Policy at the University of Dundee. From 1987 to 1991 he was a research student in the Department of Social Policy and Social Work at the University of Manchester. He spent several months in Köln in 1990, doing primary research, on the basis of which he is currently completing a doctorate in comparative health politics.

Eleanor Goldman is Associate Specialist in the Katherine Dormandy Haemostasis and Thrombosis Unit at the Royal Free Hospital, London. She is involved in the day-to-day clinical care of patients and their families, particularly those with HIV infection.

Rebecca Graham-Smith is a medical student at London Hospital Medical College, London. As part of an intercalated BSc in Sociology as Applied to Medicine in 1989–90, she conducted a research project on health care provision for women sex workers in London.

Mary Haour-Knipe recently coordinated the European Community's 'Assessing AIDS Prevention' work group surveying HIV/AIDS prevention activities for migrants and travellers in European countries. Besides the Swiss evaluation studies, her main research and publication focuses have been on migration and mental health, stress, family functioning, and social equity and health.

Graham Hart is Lecturer in Medical Sociology at University College and Middlesex School of Medicine, London. His research interests include sexual and injecting risk behaviours for HIV infection, and he has recently published papers on these subjects in the *British Medical Journal, AIDS* and *AIDS Care.* He is editor (with Peter Aggleton and Peter Davies) of *AIDS: Social Representations, Social Practices* (Falmer, 1989), *AIDS: Individual, Cultural and Policy Dimensions* (Falmer, 1990) and *AIDS: Responses, Interventions and Care* (Falmer, 1991).

Janet Holland is Research Lecturer in the Department of Policy Studies, Institute of Education, London. Her general research interests are in the area of gender, youth and class. Her current research is into young women's sexuality with the Women, Risk and AIDS Project, and the evaluation of street drug agencies.

Roger Ingham is Senior Lecturer in the Department of Psychology at the University of Southampton, where he is also Deputy Director of the Institute for Health Policy Studies. He is currently directing the ESRC funded project on Social Aspects of Risk-reduction in the Light of the Threat of HIV Infection, and has a close involvement with the World Health Organisation's Global Programme on AIDS. Other current research interests include young drivers and accident potential, and the quality of life in people with learning difficulties. Previous research interests have included football 'hooliganism' and psychological aspects of leisure. He is a past editor of *Leisure Studies.*

Susan Kippax is Head of the Macquarie University AIDS Research Unit, a unit of the National Centre for HIV Social Research. She has worked on research projects concerning the social aspects of the prevention of AIDS and has published journal articles on changes in sexual practice and sexual negotiation. She is Associate Professor in Social Psychology in the School of Behavioural Sciences at Macquarie University and has recently completed a study of the social construction of emotion (with June Crawford and others), *Emotion and Gender: Constructing Meaning from Memory*, to be published by Sage in 1992.

Jenny Kitzinger is a lesbian feminist, currently working as a research fellow at Glasgow University. Her previous work has been in the field of NHS staffing structures, maternity services, child sexual assault and young women's sexuality.

Hilary Klee is Senior Lecturer in Psychology at Manchester Polytechnic. She has directed projects concerned with HIV-related risk behaviour among injecting drug users in the North West of England. Her current research investigates the social and sexual lifestyles of amphetamine users and the risk behaviour of users of multiple drugs. She has published recently on these topics in the *British Journal of Education, AIDS Care* and the *Journal of Community and Applied Social Psychology*.

Kathy McCann is working as a social scientist in the Assessment of Health Care Needs Division at the Northern Regional Health Authority in Newcastle Upon Tyne. She has recently completed a project on Gay Men's Perceptions of HIV-Related Health and Social Care and has published papers on the study in *AIDS Care, British Journal of General Practice, Journal of Advanced Nursing* and *Counselling Quarterly*.

David Miller is a research fellow at Glasgow University. His current interests are the production of HIV/AIDS media messages and the relationship between news management and audience beliefs in Northern Ireland.

Riva Miller is a qualified Family Therapist who is AIDS Counselling Coordinator and Senior Social Worker, Haemophilia Centre, Royal Free Hospital. Recent publications include chapters in D. Miller *et al.* (Eds), *The Management of AIDS Patients* (Macmillan, 1986) and J. Studd (Ed.), *Progress in Obstetrics and Gynaecology, Vol. 8* (Churchill Livingstone, 1990) and a paper in *Health and Hygiene*.

Sofi Ospina, since participating in the study reported on here, has been coordinating HIV/AIDS prevention activities among Spanish and Portuguese-speaking communities living in Switzerland for the Federal Public Health Office. Previous work has been in HIV/AIDS prevention, in health promotion and in medical anthropology in Colombia.

Caroline Ramazanoglu is Senior Lecturer in the Sociology Department, Goldsmiths' College, University of London. Her research interests are in the area of gender, race and power and methodology, and she is a member of the Women, Risk and AIDS Project team. She is author of *Feminism and the Contradictions of Oppression* (Routledge, 1989).

Pam Rodden is a Research Assistant on the SAPA and CHAP projects in the AIDS Research Unit at Macquarie University, Sydney, Australia.

Graham Scambler is Senior Lecturer in Sociology at University College and Middlesex School of Medicine, London. His research interests include the health and quality of life of women sex workers. Apart from journal articles, his recent publications include *Sociological Theory and Medical Sociology* (Ed., Tavistock, 1987), *Epilepsy* (Tavistock, 1989) and *Sociology as Applied to Medicine*, 3rd ed. (Ed., Bailliere Tindall, 1991).

Sue Scott is Lecturer in the Sociology Department, University of Manchester, and Director of CRISAH, Centre for Research into Social Aspects of Health. A member of the Women, Risk and AIDS Project team, her other major research interests are in feminist methodology, the application of sociology to evaluation, and the sociology of mind, body and emotions.

Sue Sharpe is a freelance writer and researcher, currently working with the Women, Risk and AIDS Project team. Her main research interests are the lives and experiences of young women, and her books include *Just Like a Girl* (Penguin, 1976), *Falling for Love* (Virago, 1987) and *Voices from Home* (Virago, 1990).

David Silverman is Professor of Sociology at Goldsmiths' College, University of London. Recent publications include *Qualitative Methodology and Sociology* (Gower, 1985). *Communication and Medical Practice* (Sage, 1987) and (with J. Gubrium, eds) *The Politics of Field Research*. He has published extensively on HIV/AIDS counselling.

Karen Stenner is a researcher in the field of sexuality, young people and HIV/AIDS. At the time the chapter was written she was Research Assistant for the Southampton-based project on social aspects of risk reduction among young people. Recently published papers from the project can be found in the *Journal of Community and Applied Social Psychology* and *Health Education: Theory and Practice*.

Rachel Thomson is Research Assistant in the Sociology Department, University of Manchester. She is currently doing research into young women's sexuality for the Women, Risk and AIDS Project and completing an MA in applied social research.

Lex Watson is Senior Lecturer in Government at the University of Sydney and a Board Member of the AIDS Council of New South Wales.

Peter Weatherburn is a Senior Research Fellow for Project SIGMA (Socio-sexual Investigations of Gay Men and AIDS), working at South Bank Polytechnic. His main research interests are bisexuality and the effects of alcohol and other psychoactive drugs on HIV risk behaviour.

Alison Woodcock is Research Fellow in the Department of Psychology, University of Southampton. She has been involved in interviewing and data analysis for an Economic and Social Research Council funded project on young people's sexual behaviour in relation to HIV infection. Publications from this project (in joint authorship with Karen Stenner and Roger Ingham) appear in *Health Education Research: Theory and Practice* and in a special issue of *Community and Applied Social Psychology* on the social dimensions of AIDS.

Erwin Zimmermann was senior medical sociologist at the Institute of Social and Preventive Medicine in Lausanne, where he was involved in several ongoing evaluation studies. His research projects and publications have been in the fields of stress, delinquency, doctor-patient relationships, drug use and coping in prisons, and public housing policy.

Index

Printed and bound by CPI Group (UK) Ltd, Croydon, CR0 4YY

17/10/2024

01775686-0014